HOW TO
AVOID
BACK
SURGERY

HOW TO AVOID
Back Surgery

CHIROPRACTIC
The Proven Method for Back Pain

by
J.C. Smith, MA, DC

Published by
Chiropractic Paradigm Systems
1103 Russell Parkway
Warner Robins, GA. 31088

For book orders, phone 1-800-336-2013

Cover design by Tim Long of *Design One*, Atlanta, GA.

Other books by the author:
A Chiropractic Paradigm
The Path to Mastery in Chiropractic

Publisher's Cataloging in Publication
(prepared by Quality Books, Inc.)

Smith, J.C. (James Charles), 1948 -
How to avoid back surgery : Chiropractic - the proven method for
back pain / by J.C. Smith.
p. cm.
Includes bibliographical references.
ISBN 0-9646206-0-X

1. Backache - Chiropractic treatment. 2. Back - Surgery - Popular
works. 3. Chiropractic. 1. Title. II. Title: Chiropractic -
the proven method for back pain.

RZ265.S64S65 1996   617.5'64
QBI95-20810

FOREWORD

Back pain is an ailment which affects 80 percent of all Americans at some point in their lives. There are a myriad of causes that have been treated with multiple intended solutions. Much of the treatment over the years how has become suspect, proven ineffective or iatrogenically causes a condition worse than the presenting back condition. The key in back pain treatment is to avoid surgery at all costs, at least until all alternative methods have been exhausted.

As a chiropractor over the past 17 years, I know better. In some respects, I know too well. I had a back surgery (clawing, kicking and screaming all the way) with a fortunate, successful outcome. I had a highly skilled surgeon operating on a definitive cause that would not respond any other way. (Also, the process was urged by my wife, as she was tired of tripping over me where I was camped on the bedroom floor for two weeks.) In other words, surgery was my last resort. For most of you who read this book, it should also be your last resort! You can beat it without surgery.

Why would I tell you to beat surgery at all costs, if mine worked? Many low back operations do not work. People often end up with intractable chronic pain, paralysis, additional surgeries, permanent disability and even death! I was one of the lucky ones.

I managed my herniated disc over nine years after my causative bicycle crash, with exercise, spinal adjustments by my chiropractor, daily attention to lifting and working properly and a positive mental attitude. Unfortunately, I fell victim to my human side and lost much of the discipline that had kept me from an irreversible surgical situation. At the height of my deconditioned state I had a minor trauma which resulted in a major problem. Regrettably, I had to place my entire life and livelihood into the hands of a neurosurgeon, the same predicament from which I had saved so many of my patients over the years. It was not an easy choice for a chiropractor, especially *this* chiropractor.

This book is about how *not* to follow the path I traveled. Hopefully, in reading this book you can keep yourself off the surgeon's table, and maintain the daily routine necessary to do so for life. Go forth, read, learn and don't become a surgical statistic.

G. Steven Baer, DC
Chiropractic Associates, Inc.
Middletown, Ohio

ACKNOWLEDGMENTS

In the production of this book, there are many people who have helped, either directly or indirectly, and to whom I would like now to give thanks.

To Christine Thompson, Esq., associate editor of the *Journal of the American Chiropractic Association*, for her editorial polish and professional feedback.

To Megan Hutnick Smith, my wife, for her love and support and, most of all, for her computer expertise, without which this computer-illiterate probably would still be writing this manuscript in longhand.

To my children, Jamie and Jackson, may the time we've lost together be recaptured with fun at the Cuckoo Clock house.

To every doctor of chiropractic who has worked tirelessly without the recognition he or she deserves, let this book be a testament that our time has finally arrived.

To my patients whose clinical problems have taught me the broad value of chiropractic care and whose support, despite the many social and economic disincentives, have shown me their commitment and appreciation, without which money alone could not have maintained me (and every DC) on this path less traveled.

Lastly, let me say to every person who suffers from back pain: Let this book help you to understand and to solve your condition without the need of drugs or unnecessary surgery by introducing you to the world of chiropractic health care. Indeed, this book may just be your first step up the learning curve to better health. Enjoy the trip!

INTRODUCTION

This book could save you untold amounts of money as well as suffering. Back pain is among the leading ailments plaguing modern society, and it's only getting worse. The costs are staggering, the suffering is epidemic, and the medical methods – drugs and surgery – just don't work well as the leading researchers now tell us. Indeed, back pain and back surgery are both facts of life that can be avoided in 99 percent of cases. This book will teach you how to do just that and much more.

As a practicing chiropractor, my heart has been heavy too many times when I witness the aftermath of unnecessary back surgery on victims whose conditions could easily have been helped with safe and effective chiropractic care – seeing a patient's life turned upside down by a failed back surgery that was never needed and which only served to further complicate the problem. To say that back surgeons have left a wake of destruction in their path is an understatement. And to watch them laugh all the way to the bank because too many insurance programs refuse to pay for chiropractic care, instead paying billions for ineffective back surgeries, is a sham that only exists in the insulated world of medical care. Most back surgeries are nothing less than professional predation hidden within the sacrosanct air of hospitals. Hopefully, this book will save you or someone you know from these medical crimes that can be avoided with chiropractic care.

I have to applaud those patients who have found their way out of the medical box of solutions. Being healthy in America is a difficult challenge, especially when it comes to back attacks. One must swim upstream against the currents of the medical profession, hospitals, drug companies and the insurance "system" which all stand to profit from unnecessary back surgeries. As you will learn, there are simple reasons why back surgeries are epidemic and why they fail to solve this problem anyway. Let me also say that I take my hat off to the millions of patients who have found the courage to resist the bigotry and propaganda of the medical system and who have selected the chiropractic solution to the ageless problem of back pain.

I also want to take my hat off to the thousands of doctors of chiropractic who have fought for a century to bring a new model of health care to the American public. Fighting one of the most powerful forces in our country, the American Medical Association (AMA) is a task few alternative health professions have withstood. Despite the many setbacks, the chiropractic method has survived and now is being hailed by experts as the best solution to this back pain epidemic. Without their dedication to the chiropractic principle and their belief in the basic American right of freedom of choice, doctors of chiropractic long ago would have succumbed to the dirty tricks of our medical detractors, thus denying the chiropractic solution to the public. Consequently, the epidemic of back surgeries could have been much worse if it weren't for the courage of chiropractors.

I believe it's time for Americans to give thanks for the perseverance and dedication of these chiropractic professionals who have, for over a century, overcome medical prejudice, institutional discrimination, public stigmas and governmental apathy in their quest to bring a new idea to the fight against pain and disease. After reading this book, you can show your newly found appreciation by visiting a chiropractic office to learn more about this effective science.

However, let me warn you: If you decide not to follow the advice in this book and ignore proven spinal care methods now recommended by experts, your unfortunate fate awaits – the great possibility of failed back surgery and a life of permanent disability. It's your choice to make an informed decision once you've studied the facts on chiropractic and back surgery. Hopefully you'll chose the right path – chiropractic spinal care.

Once you understand the dynamics of this healing art, the benefits of improved health will speak loudly – especially if that includes avoiding back surgery. Believe me when I tell you there is more to solving spinal problems than simply more drugs and more surgeries. Let a professional chiropractor introduce you to a new world of good health, naturally. It will be one of the most important decisions of your life, just as it has been for millions of people who have turned to chiropractic care.

Yours in Health,
J.C. Smith, DC
Warner Robins, Georgia USA

Table of Contents

CHIROPRACTIC

The
Proven Method
for
Back Pain

CHAPTER ONE

How to Avoid Back Surgery

*"Anyone who has a back surgery
without seeing a chiropractor first
should also have his head examined."*
– Robert Mendelsohn, MD
Author, *Confessions of a Medical Heretic*

If you want to avoid back surgery, go to a chiropractor. It's that simple. The newest scientific research verifies that for America's number one health problem – back pain – chiropractic spinal care has proven the most effective treatment. As one investigator, Pran Manga, PhD simply put it, "The evidence is overpowering."[1]

I know some people may flinch at this suggestion, inasmuch as some medical doctors have ridiculed chiropractic care to discourage patients with their professional slander. Yes, I realize that some reporters in the written and electronic media also have infected the public with half-truths and anecdotal scare stories about chiropractic. Yes, I am quite aware of patients' fears, worries and concerns – real or imagined. Believe me, after two decades of practicing chiropractic, I think I've heard it all. Yet, the fact remains, if you want to avoid back surgery and stop the pain of a back attack, I urge you to consider chiropractic care. Despite the old misunderstandings, the facts are now clear: Chiropractic care is the best solution to the vast majority of back pain problems.

Although Dr. Robert Mendelsohn's quote may seem rather insulting to the many people who already have succumbed to back surgery, his sentiments are painfully honest. Patients should first seek chiropractic care because it can help over 90 percent of all back pain problems. Yes, there are the exceptions that require medical care – the fractures, cancers and pathologies, and the rare cases of true disc ruptures that strike less than one percent of all cases. Yes, a few patients will feel better after a lumbar fusion or discectomy, not knowing that they possibly could have felt better without surgery if they had tried chiropractic first. Yes, there are some patients who tried chiropractic care, got poor results for whatever reasons, and went to a surgeon who helped them. But for the most part, the research has shown that for the vast majority of back pain cases, chiropractic is the safest, most clinically-effective and least expensive method to manage this epidemic.

I also agree with Dr. Mendelsohn's belief that some people do need to have their heads examined when it comes to their concepts of chiropractic care. It always amazes me when patients with failed back surgeries come to my office seeking care and they didn't try chiropractic first. When I ask them why they didn't, many reply that they were afraid to ask their MD to refer for fear of ridicule;

some, unbelievably, were afraid of spinal adjustments because the surgeon told them chiropractic might paralyze them! Incredibly, some people are more afraid of simple, gentle spinal manipulation than going under the knife! That fear, however unwarranted is nevertheless a part of the problem in convincing people that chiropractic care should be their first avenue for back pain treatment. If Dr. Mendelsohn were to examine the minds of patients who have undergone back surgery without seeking chiropractic care first, he would find as I have, that the public's perception of this great healing art mostly is filled with untruths from medical misinformation.

For over 100 years chiropractors have been helping millions of people avoid disabling back pain and ineffective back surgeries, yet the medical world continues to mislead its patients about the underlying cause of back pain and clinical benefits of spinal manipulative therapy. Indeed, it's next to impossible for most patients to find the truth about this serious epidemic of back pain because of the medical misinformation, insurance disincentives, unethical medical doctors and the general lack of the public's understanding about what is the actual cause of most back pain. The more you learn about back pain, the more you will realize that most often it is not caused by disc problems, which has been the major claim of the medical world, nor is surgery the most effective cure. It's my goal to help you, the 80 percent of adults who will experience a serious back attack sometime in their lifetime, to understand the nature of back pain and the best remedy for this pervasive problem.

The Medical Explanations of Back Pain

For decades, whenever patients complained of back pain, the medical professionals automatically diagnosed the cause as either a "pulled muscle" or a disc problem – a "ruptured," "herniated," "degenerated" or "slipped" disc. Today we can honestly say that neither of these beliefs have withstood the scrutiny of research investigators. As you will learn, recent research studies with MRI exams by orthopedic surgeons have proven the abnormal disc premise to be very suspect. Simply, they found that most back pain has little to do with disc abnormalities or pulled muscles. They did conclude that the high failure rate of back surgery is due primarily to these false claims that still predominate in the medical world, despite the modern research that undermines these mistaken beliefs that have lead to millions of mismanaged patients and an epidemic of failed back surgeries.

Not only are too many back surgeries performed, the experts found there are too many expensive MRI exams routinely prematurely performed on back pain patients. Moreover, they found routine misinterpretations of MRI exams that are mistakenly used to convince patients of the need for surgery when, in fact, they may not require it. In other words, just because an MRI exam is "positive" for some type of disc abnormality, it doesn't mean it is the source of pain, nor is surgery required to fix it. While some MDs would argue this point, recent medical research verifies that most back pain has little to do with disc problems.

2

Perhaps the most shocking report in the U.S. on this issue has surfaced with two separate studies. In 1994 *The New England Journal of Medicine* published a report which as picked up by the Associated Press titled: "Ruptured Discs Not Always a Pain – Research suggests too much emphasis is placed on them." The study was conducted on 98 healthy volunteers by Maureen C. Jensen, MD, and colleagues from Hoag Memorial Hospital in Newport Beach, California. Of the 98 asymptomatic patients, "52 percent had a bulge at least at one level, 27 percent had a protrusion, and one percent had an extrusion. Thirty-eight percent had an abnormality of more than one intervertebral disc."[2] This study roughly duplicated a study completed four years earlier by Scott Boden, MD, an orthopedic surgeon at Emory University in Atlanta.[3] Their conclusions shocked the medical community by criticizing the basic routines widely used by medical doctors:

> "The MRI should never be used as a screening test, which is unfortunately the way it is very commonly used today," Boden said. "In fact, use of the MRI too early in somebody's disease process can result in seeing these findings that are like gray hair – everybody gets them – and can result in over-treatment... The Jensen study suggests that disc peculiarities [bulges, herniations, protrusions] 'may frequently be coincidental' in people with back trouble. <u>In other words, the disc might not be the cause of the pain. And if so, fixing it is a waste.</u>"

This misleading medical premise that most all back pain is due to disc problems has lead to an epidemic of back surgeries in the United States that is unparalleled in the world – American surgeons do five times more back surgeries than any other country in the world. Of the 300,000 disc surgeries done each year for ruptured discs, medical authority B.E. Finneson, PhD, admits that 50 to 90 percent are unnecessary and ineffective. Moreover, his statistics showed that over 53 percent of these patients are in the same pain or worse than before their surgeries![4]

Many contemporary researchers now believe that the disc premise as the cause of back pain may actually be greatly exaggerated. For instance, extensive research done by W.H. Kirkaldy-Willis, MD, and David Cassidy, DC indicates that discs are involved in <u>fewer than 10 percent</u> of back pain cases.[6] Nikolai Bogduk, MD, PhD in his text, *Clinical Anatomy of the Lumbar Spine,* states that discs are involved in <u>fewer than 5 percent</u> of these cases.[7] Moreover, in his article published in *Spine* magazine, V. Mooney, MD writes that he believes it is <u>less than 1 percent.</u>[8] Objective research disproves the medical emphasis that disc abnormalities are the root cause of back pain and supports the belief that disc surgery is, as Dr. Boden believes, a waste of time, money and effort.

The mistaken emphasis on discs has created an epidemic of surgical failures and has cost over $75 billion a year in our country alone and over $100 billion worldwide. This is a huge problem that has been mismanaged for decades and has cost billions for rather poor results. As the RAND Corporation Report, "The Appropriateness of Spinal Manipulation for Low-Back Pain," in 1992 stated:

> "As health-care costs continue to climb and as evidence mounts that some

medical and surgical procedures are overused, there is a growing perception that the United States is not receiving sufficient value for its expenditures on health... This underlying uncertainty about how to treat certain diseases may be in part responsible for overuse and for the needless expenditures and risk such inappropriate use places on payers and patients."[9]

If you want to avoid the expense of being a victim of the ineffective surgical approach to back pain, I urge you to re-think what you've been told is the basic cause of your problem. You might be shocked to find that your so-called "slipped disc" hasn't really slipped nor is it the primary cause of your pain and that back surgery may not be as successful as your surgeon leads you to believe. For example, one Workers' Compensation study in Washington state indicated that lumbar fusions had a success rate of only 23 percent, which means 77 percent were considered failures![10] Although they confirmed the presence of abnormal discs on examination, the surgeries failed to ease the patients' pain in most cases because discs were not the main source of pain. Hospitals now require patients to sign an informed consent before they are blindly lead into this expensive and risky surgery. Hopefully, someone will inform these patients that chiropractic care is now recommended before any back surgery.

So the million (or should I say $100 billion) dollar question remains: If "slipped discs" and "pulled muscles" are not the causes of most back pain, what is?" That's exactly what the U.S. Public Health Service wondered when its Agency for Health Care Policy and Research (AHCPR) conducted its two-year study of over 4,000 articles on acute low back pain in adults.[11] Its recommendations shocked the medical world as much as had Drs. Jensen and Boden's research. The agency concluded that only one in 100 back surgeries is helpful, which was a nice way of saying 99 percent of back surgeries are unnecessary. This panel of 23 medical experts recommended that spinal manipulation is the best initial form of professional treatment for most cases of back pain, shocking the press, the public, and most of all, the medical world. If disc abnormalities are not the cause of most back pain, and if spinal manipulation is the best initial form of treatment, then what causes this enormous problem that affects 80 percent of all adults at sometime during their lives?

The answer to this billion dollar question is: "Spinal joints." Simply put: Discs don't slip, but joints do! Few people understand that the vast majority of back pain is caused by misalignment of the 137 joints in the spinal column. As you will learn, this fact explains why the U.S. Public Health Service now recommends spinal manipulation as the best initial form of professional treatment for acute low back pain in adults. The AHCPR guideline contained other recommendations that your local MD would probably never tell you about – that the standard medical approach of pain pills, muscle relaxants, ultrasound, traction and many other traditional physical therapies are now consider temporary at best, expensive and ineffective for long term benefits, and that only one in 200 low back problems present a dangerous condition requiring expensive testing like an MRI, CT exam or myelogram. In fact, it is very difficult to get to the truth about the best form of

4

treatment for back problems if you listen only to the medical professionals.

Indeed, the real challenge is to learn the facts about the cause of most back pain, to learn about the benefits of chiropractic spinal care and to accept the responsibility to implement a few basic hygienic habits to help avoid back attacks and surgery by maintaining good spinal health. This challenge presents a lot for the average person to comprehend and demands that he or she adapt to new concepts, new attitudes and new daily lifestyle habits. After caring for thousands of patients with back attacks and failed back surgery, I have concluded that the average patient fails to understand his or her problem, wants only a quick-fix, and generally ignores the problem until it occurs again. That's equivalent of a dental patient who ignores toothpaste, flossing and periodic check-ups, waits for the inevitable toothache, only seeks a quick-fix from the dentist, and then continues to ignore preventative care to avoid relapses. We know that this approach doesn't work for dental health care, nor does it work for spinal health care. Unfortunately, the public has little understanding of preventative spinal care to avoid the inevitable back attacks that the majority of adults will suffer during their lives.

The solution to the back pain epidemic is not just substituting chiropractic care for back surgeries, although that is an excellent starting point recommended by the new federal guideline on acute low back pain in adults. The real challenge is to modify your lifestyle to incorporate new habits that work to prevent the attack in the first place and to rehab the weakened spinal area to avoid a relapse. Just as Americans are very aware about their dental hygiene, I believe the same level of awareness about their spinal health will be the best solution to this problem of back pain. Unfortunately, most people know more about their teeth and take better care of them than they do about their spines, even though the spine is vastly more important than teeth. A simple remedy that I preach to my patients is to take a "dental attitude" about your spine – regular preventative measures with periodic check-ups.

My goal as a practitioner is to teach my patients these preventative measures as I treat their back pain; otherwise a relapse is certain. And, as *informed* patients, most people also learn there's more to chiropractic care than just achieving back pain relief. But for now, if your goal is to avoid back surgery or to avoid a relapse of back pain, it starts with your understanding some basic facts about your spinal column, which remains a puzzle to most people. Let the latest research from international experts explain the causes of back pain and the best method to correct this epidemic. Don't just take my word on it. As a practicing chiropractor, I have studied this issue for over 20 years and I have taken care of thousands of patients – satisfied chiropractic patients as well as dissatisfied medical failures, those poor souls who tried the medical model and regretted it later. Even though I can say I speak from valid experiences, don't take my word alone on this important issue. Let the researchers from around the world convince you to the validity of chiropractic care. As you learn more about your spine and how it works, you too will conclude, as these researchers have, that chiropractic spinal care is the best solution for the majority of back pain problems.

CHAPTER TWO

The Dilemma of Back Pain

"Low back pain is a 20th century health-care disaster."
– Gordon Waddell, MD
Researcher and Professor of Orthopaedic Surgery,
Western Infirmary, Glasglow, Scotland

What do you say to someone who had a back surgery that didn't help and was probably never needed? What would you tell a disabled patient with permanent back pain from an ineffective surgery that was based on a false premise and an incorrect diagnosis? What do you say to someone stoned on useless pain pills and muscle relaxants and who is still in pain? How do you help a skeptical patient who now is afraid to have spinal adjustments because he was frightened by unethical MDs who knowingly lied about chiropractic care? How do you console someone who realizes he was mislead about his back problem and now is angry at the world? What would you say?

Would you tell him that he is a just one small part of a 20th century health-care disaster that costs the country billions each year? Would you tell him to sue the surgeon who slandered chiropractic care and who profited from an incorrect diagnosis and failed back surgery? Would you tell him that according to the U.S. Public Health Service report on acute low back pain only one in 100 back surgeries is helpful? Would you tell him the truth about his dilemma – that he was misdiagnosed, misinformed and mistreated?

Would you tell him that if there's any hope to help his back pain it rests with the very care that he has been scared of – chiropractic adjustments? Would you tell him that his failed surgery is *water under the bridge* and, unless he wants to have more pain, more relapses and possibly more surgeries, he had better sober up to a new reality and learn how to stabilize his weakened spine with a lot of work, time and lifestyle changes? Would you tell him that there is still hope, even though the high-tech wonders of modern medicine have failed him miserably?

This tragic situation is one that doctors of chiropractic encounter every day in this country. Back problems debilitate thousands of people in the U.S. every year, and considering acute low back pain strikes 80 percent of all adults sometime, your chance of facing this very dilemma is greater than you think. According to the U.S. Department of Health and Human Services, each year about 34 million Americans – approximately 20 percent of the adult population – suffers from back problems.[1] In any given month, 41.7 percent of women and 34.5 percent of men in the United States experience low back pain.[2] In fact, back pain is growing at an epidemic rate, and only seems to be getting worse as our country becomes more deconditioned by its affluent, sedentary lifestyle.

Compounding this high prevalence rate of back pain is the sad realization of the epidemic of failed back surgeries, a disaster for thousands of unfortunate victims of unnecessary back surgery. "Many patients with lower back pain are overtreated," according to David C. Lanier, MD, of the U.S. Public Health Service. "Patients are given too much medication, too much bed rest, and too much surgery."[3] While Dr. Lanier's admission is forthright, it fails to address the magnitude of this pervasive problem in terms of costs and human suffering – a situation that has been glossed over by the medical establishment for decades.

This tragedy is best told by a chiropractor who is in the unique position of helping these medical failures as the proverbial "last resort." This is a story that every person needs to hear because back pain is a problem that most everyone inevitably faces sometime in his or her life. Considering the present confusing state of affairs in the area of back pain treatments, proper care for back pain is a dilemma that few people can avoid and a dilemma that needs new answers.

Actually, this dilemma may strike close to home and may already have faced you or someone you know. Who doesn't know someone who has had a failed back surgery? Most often everyone has a family member or a friend who has been a victim, and most of them are rarely any better. Indeed, you have an important decision to make, and the more accurate information you have about back pain, chiropractic care and back surgery, the better able you will be to make an informed decision. You can avoid the tragic scenario of a failed back surgery for yourself if you make the right choice now – it is an important decision that will affect you the rest of your life, just as it did me and others suffering from the inevitable back attacks that strike millions of people every day.

I recall the moment when I was forced to face this dilemma as a patient. During my collegiate football days at the University of California at Berkeley, I was tackled once by a rather large defensive end. I awoke 20 minutes later with a slight concussion and found I could not move my back without extreme pain. The team doctor, an orthopedic surgeon, told me I had a "slipped disc" and needed back surgery. My roommate, who suffered from low back pain and sciatica (leg pain), told me I should see his chiropractor instead. This dilemma -- choosing between an MD and a DC for back pain – is a problem that most all Americans will face sometime during their lives.

Who is best qualified to treat back pain is the center of a controversy that is confusing for many people. For decades the medical profession dominated this field by offering drugs and surgery as weapons in their arsenal to fight back pain. Outside the medical box, chiropractors have brought to Americans a natural alternative – spinal adjustments – to combat the massive problem of back pain. The argument whether back surgeries or spinal adjustments work best to solve this epidemic has been the focus of much scientific research during the last decade, and the findings have finally answered this dilemma. According to John J. Triano, DC, the staff chiropractor at The Texas Back Institute and a member of the panel of 23 experts of the AHCPR report, "When used within the first month of symptoms, spinal manipulation has been shown to be effective."[4]

In fact, the much beleaguered chiropractic profession now has been vindicated by the recent research coming from many prestigious sources which has proven that spinal manipulation is the best treatment for the vast majority of back problems. In essence, this new research says, "Back surgeries are OUT and spinal manipulation is IN."

Back Pain – America's Largest Epidemic

Do you realize that more people suffer from back pain than any other major ailment? Over 80 percent of adults will experience a low back problem sometime in their lives, whereas only 50 percent of Americans will suffer a heart attack and 33 percent will develop cancer. Back pain always has been a major problem afflicting all civilizations, but mostly it has been ignored because it is not considered a life-threatening problem like cancer or heart disease. Nevertheless, back pain is now the number one disabling condition for people under the age of 45, and it is the second cause of disability for those over 45, other than heart disease. While back pain may not be an immediate threat to your life, it is obviously a serious obstacle to your well-being and livelihood. In fact, today back pain statistically is America's number one health problem, afflicting more people than any other health condition.

It also has become a very expensive problem, costing over $75 billion in the U.S. alone in direct medical costs and indirect costs associated with lost productivity. When wage replacement, retraining, retirement, disability and other expenses are added, the total can cost employers as much as $100 billion annually, according to an extensive 1995 study by Metropolitan Life Insurance Company, Health and Safety Education Division, Medical Department. Other shocking statistics about back pain reveal: It is the most frequently reported health reason for absence among all workers; the average physician and hospital charges to MetLife for each back surgery in 1993 totaled just under $14,000; for non-surgical back problem the average total charge per case was $7,120; and the number of back and disc surgeries in the U.S. was 22.5 percent higher in 1992 than in 1990.[5]

Another study in 1993 on the cost of treating low back pain from Liberty Mutual Insurance Company's records found that low back pain cases represented 16 percent of all their claims and accounted for 33 percent of all their claim costs. Their average claim was $8,321 for low back pain. The most expensive states for low back pain treatment was Texas ($17,714), Massachusetts ($14,516), Louisiana ($12,928), Connecticut ($12,424) and Washington D.C., ($12,126). The least expensive states were Indiana ($2,684), Wisconsin ($3,774), Utah ($3,808), Delaware ($3,870) and Nebraska ($3,848).[6]

Not only is back pain epidemic and expensive, but the medical mismanagement of back pain is now being highly criticized as ineffective, costly and causing more harm than good in many cases. The standard recipe of medical ingredients for the diagnosis and treatment of back pain just hasn't proven clinically-effective and has lead researchers to new conclusions about solving this costly epidemic.

Considering these facts, it is obvious why orthopedist Dr. Gordon Waddell said, "Low back pain is a 20th century health-care disaster."[7]

In response to this crisis, during the past few years, the U.S. Public Health Service, the Ontario (Canada) Ministry of Health and the British government, to name but a few of the many countries investigating this epidemic of back pain, all have concluded that chiropractic management has proven more effective than medical methods for the vast majority of mechanical low back pain problems. When compared directly with medical methods, chiropractic spinal care was found to be twice as effective in many studies, and the cost was also found to be a fraction of the typical medical management of drugs and surgery. In summary, chiropractic care was determined to be safer, quicker, cheaper and more clinically-effective for this epidemic of back pain. As Dr. Pran Manga stated after his research review for the Ontario (Canada) Ministry of Health, there was a "constellation of evidence" endorsing chiropractic care for the treatment of low back pain.[8]

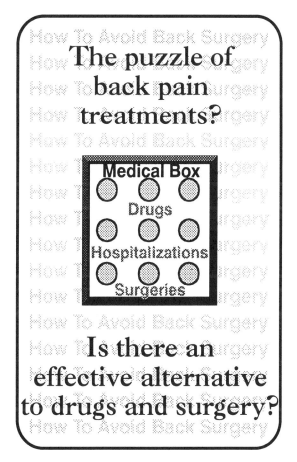

The research also has repeatedly shown that the medical premise that most back pain is due to disc derangements is very questionable and over-stated, and the medical treatments – pain pills, muscle relaxants and disc surgery -- also have proven clinically ineffective. Indeed, one British study concluded that medical mismanagement has actually contributed to, rather than solved this epidemic of back problems and escalating costs. Her Majesty's Stationary Office in London in its *Report of a Clinical Standards Advisory Group Committee on Back Pain* states: "Traditional medical treatment has failed to halt this epidemic and may even have contributed to it. There is a clear need to reconsider our whole approach to the management of low back pain and disability."[9] The idea that low back pain is a 20th century health-care disaster stems not so much from the high prevalence of back pain, as much as it stems from the grossly ineffective medical management of these cases. As you will learn, the medical approach of drugs and surgery has failed to halt or improve this epidemic of back pain, and it actually is now considered to be one of the main causes of this huge dilemma.

While this news may have shocked the public and the medical profession alike, it has been sweet music to the chiropractic profession which has struggled for over a century to bring another perspective to the growing problem of back pain. Despite medical opposition at every turn, the chiropractic profession has fought to give the public freedom of choice in its treatment options. The chiropractic choice now has proven the most effective treatment for America's number one health-care problem. For many victims of failed back surgery, this new research and revelations about chiropractic care may be too late, but for many others, this book may help them avoid unnecessary drugs and back surgeries that have mostly added to the massive epidemic of back disabilities.

Not So "Alternative" Anymore

Chiropractic was once considered mainly an underground health-care profession working on the fringes of respectability. Now, new light has revealed that "alternative" medicine is on the rise. *The New England Journal of Medicine* reported a 1990 study entitled "Unconventional Medicine in the United States," by David Eisenberg, MD, et al.[10] The results stunned the medical establishment when they revealed that one-third of all Americans sought care from alternative doctors and therapists. Not only did these Americans seek alternative care from the mainstream medical doctors, they actually made 425 million visits to chiropractors, massage therapists, acupuncturists, and nutritionists, among others. This huge number shocked the medical establishment because during the same period, patients utilized MDs for 388 million visits. Apparently "alternative" isn't so alternative anymore!

Another interesting fact about these Americans using unconventional health-care was that the majority were college-educated, upper-middle class consumers. These patients were not uninformed, uneducated subjects naively being lead by scam artists, as some would have you believe. These were patients who made informed decisions to seek care that they believed would best solve their health needs. Not only were there more office visits to non-MD practitioners, in 1990 these patients also spent comparable out-of-pocket money – $10.3 billion – to see non-MDs, compared to $12.8 billion for all hospitalizations. Despite insurance discrimination, people are willing to pay for this natural health care themselves. The most common ailments reported by these patients were for back pain, headaches, insomnia, anxiety and depression. Apparently, many Americans have learned that not all health problems can be solved with drugs and surgery; they are willing to pay for natural methods despite the lack of medical insurance coverage.

The Eisenberg study also revealed another startling revelation: The high usage of chiropractic was a well kept secret in health care because few patients were willing to discuss their alternative care with their MDs. Apparently, these patients either felt it was none of their MD's business or they were afraid to tell him or her. Many people are discouraged by stupid remarks some MDs make to patients even after seeing the positive results chiropractic care has brought them.

As a practicing doctor of chiropractic, I understand why these patients didn't tell their MDs – they just didn't want to be insulted and ridiculed; moreover, many patients are frightened by unethical surgeons who use a *voo-doo* diagnosis to scare patients away from chiropractors.

Let me explain a *voo-doo* diagnosis, because you may have been a victim of this unethical ploy. When failed medical patients finally come into my office as a last resort, I always ask them why they didn't try chiropractic first. Most of the time they had asked their surgeon if they should try chiropractic before surgery, but the surgeon did his best version of a *voo-doo* diagnosis to scare the hell out of the unsuspecting patient. Often the MD has stated, *"If you don't have my surgery, you'll get worse. And if you let a chiropractor touch you, he'll paralyze you."* For most uninformed patients, this slanderous statement is enough to scare them into a useless surgery.

In fact, a recent study confirmed that the main sources of chiropractic horror stories is the medical profession. Cheryl Hawk, DC, PhD, and her associates completed a study on perceived barriers to chiropractic utilization using focus groups. The participants were people who had suffered back pain but had never visited a chiropractor. All the participants were asked, *"Have you ever considered seeking chiropractic care for your back pain?"* and if so, *"How did you ultimately decide not to see a chiropractor?"* Medical doctors were the primary source of the horror stories that deterred participants from seeking chiropractic care. In fact, in one community closely linked to activities of a medical school and teaching hospital, focus group participants more often expressed fear of chiropractors than did people living in other communities. The media was a second source, particularly the 1995 report on chiropractic that aired on ABC's news program, *"20/20."*[11]

It is shocking to hear how low some surgeons will stoop to convince a patient to undergo an unnecessary surgery. And it never ceases to amaze me how some patients are scared to get a simple, painless spinal adjustment, but not a risky and expensive back surgery. It must take quite a bit of deception on the part of these *voo-doo* surgeons to implant the idea that chiropractic adjustments hurt or are dangerous. In fact, chiropractors have the lowest malpractice rates of any health professionals. The insurance companies know who is hurting whom, and they know that chiropractic adjustments are extremely safe. Every doctor wishes his method had a one in a million iatrogenic rate. Yet, some MDs tell patients just the opposite to lure them into unnecessary surgery.

According to Andrew Weil, MD, "Patients correctly sense that doctors are going to make fun of them or 'punish' them for using these other modalities. People are discouraged by the expense, risk (of drug and surgical side-effects) and lack of effectiveness of regular medicine." The medical men now are learning what the public has finally learned as well – that drugs and surgery, the main tools of the medical profession, cannot solve all health problems, especially spinal problems. According to their publication, *The Trends Journal,* the prestigious Trends Research Institute "forecasts continued mainstreaming of alternative treatments such as chiropractic, acupuncture, ayurveda and other non-allopathic interventions."

Ironically, these experts often talk as if these methods are just now here to stay, not realizing that many of them have been here far longer than most medical methods. As Congressman Dana Rohrabacher (R-Calif.) stated after the release of the AHCPR guideline on low back pain, "It only took them *umteen* years to discover that chiropractic care is effective... when we have millions of Americans who discovered that a long time ago, and are living healthier, happier lives because of it." Unfortunately, due to the obstructionist position of political medicine, many millions of other Americans have been discouraged from benefiting from chiropractic care, much to their own chagrin. Hopefully the new guideline will encourage patients to overcome these medical deterrents and enjoy living healthier, happier lives as Congressman Rohrabacher mentioned.

In his book, *The Assault on Medical Freedom*, author P. Joseph Lisa succinctly summarized the unfair methods used by political medicine to discredit its competition:

> "Alternative medicine should complement allopathic medicine. In some cases there is a need for allopathic medicine. In other cases it would be best to employ some form of alternative (or complementary) medicine. In some instances, a patient may require a combination of approaches to healing. However, for any one discipline to sit in official judgment of its economic competitors and to distribute propaganda to the public about how bad its competitors' remedies and treatments are is not only unethical, it is bad medicine. It is unfair and illegal, in that it violates the Sherman Antitrust Act which forbids such anti-competitive activity. Regrettably, restraint of trade, unfair trade practices, anti-competitive activity, and conspiracy to eliminate the competition have been hallmarks of American medicine. It has been this way from its inception and blatantly continues to this day."[12]

Obviously, the medical world is not pleased about the increasing popularity of chiropractic and other natural health-care professions. According to Dr. Andrew Weil, advocate of alternative health care, "It's going to send a ripple of shock through the medical community. A large number of patient dollars are being lost to unconventional therapies." His comment reflects the thought that greater clinical effectiveness of "unconventional therapies" is not the main concern in this trend to use non-MDs, as much as is the main problem of their lost revenues.

The medical monopoly controls every aspect of health care in this country and has been the greatest obstruction to any real health care reform. According to the Cato Institute, a public policy research foundation in Washington, DC, in its monograph titled, "The Medical Monopoly: Protecting Consumers or Limiting Competition?", federal and insurance regulations influenced by the AMA are believed to be the main contributing factors in the spiraling costs of health care:

> "Any serious reform of the U.S. health care system must address the medical monopoly. Barriers to entry into the health care marketplace are partially

responsible for high health costs and lack of access to primary and preventative health care...nearly all economists recognize that professional licensure laws act as a barrier to entry that decreases competition and increases price....Accordingly, individuals should have the legal right to decide with whom they will contract for the provision and coordination of their health care services: doctors, mid-wives, nurse practitioners, chiropractors...Any restriction denies Americans the right to make decisions about their own bodies."[13]

Indeed, the increasing use of non-MD practitioners by the public "should raise a red flag for all of us," according to M. Roy Schwarz, MD, senior vice president for medical education and science at the American Medical Association. Obviously, Dr. Schwarz's main concern is not the ineffectiveness of medical care that drives patients elsewhere to seek help, instead he mainly is concerned with potential lost revenues. He particularly is concerned that patients rarely discuss their alternative treatments with their physician, creating a communication gap that leads to an incomplete picture of care. According to Dr. Schwarz, "It says that people are willing to experiment." As I see it, although Dr. Schwarz's viewpoint is understandable, it is really no experiment to rely on safe and natural methods of healing which have, in many instances, existed longer than modern drugs and surgeries. In fact, the real experiments in treatment are the so-called "wonder" drugs and the unnecessary surgeries that predominate in today's medical world. Perhaps people now are seeking to correct the underlying causes of their health problems with natural methods instead of masking the symptoms, as the fascination with drugs and surgeries often does. Perhaps people finally have realized that the "wonder" drugs aren't so wonderful after all and they are willing to take charge of their own health decisions without the intervention or blessings of their medical doctors.

Julian Whitaker, MD a medical whistleblower who has been very critical of the traditional medical "drug 'em, cut 'em" methods and switched instead to natural health-care methods, wrote in his *Health & Healing* newsletter in November 1994:

"Can you name any therapy commonly used in conventional medicine that is NOT a prescription drug or surgical procedure? I bet not... It's not that safe alternative treatments don't exist – they do... But most conventional doctors believe anything other than prescription drugs or surgery has no benefit in the treatment or prevention of disease. This belief is absurd... Conventional doctors claim to have superior knowledge. However, their knowledge is so restricted by negative bias that many are perpetrators of disease, rather than healers. This "anti-supplement" [and anti-chiropractic] climate also dictates that true breakthroughs in nutritional science which could save millions of lives are ignored – or condemned."[14]

It is a sad situation when patients are afraid to ask their medical doctor about natural methods of healing that may be more effective, safer and less costly. People have learned that there are apparently *right* and *wrong* ways to get well, especially if they do not use drugs and surgery. Political medicine has fought long and hard to deny patients freedom of choice in health care, despite the obvious shortcomings of its own methods. Inasmuch as Americans in 1994 spent over one trillion dollars for health care and, considering the fact that we lead the world in every category of chronic degenerative disease, a case can easily be made that Americans are not getting their money's worth in health care. And so-called experts wonder why people are seeking safer, cheaper and more effective "alternatives" without input from MDs? Go figure!

Don't Be Afraid To Ask

This book is intended for those open-minded people who have been hesitant to use a chiropractor because they were afraid to ask, or who perhaps just aren't sure – they just don't know enough about this profession in order to make an informed decision. Hopefully, reading this book will stimulate you to seek alternatives to many medical procedures. You may find, as have one-third of all Americans, that alternative health care offers many safe and effective solutions to health needs. Although chiropractic care offers the most effective answer to America's number one health problem – the epidemic of back pain – it also treats many other non-back pain conditions. And combined with proper nutrition, vitamin supplementation, aerobic recreation and other innovative natural methods, many people are finding the answers to their health needs in the world of natural health care.

But please don't feel you have to give up medicine in order to become a chiropractic patient. Many MDs have used this type of ultimatum to deny treatment options to their patients. Chiropractic's aim is not to eliminate medicine at all – that would be impossible and is a ridiculous notion – nor is it opposed to all drugs and surgeries. As a whole, chiropractic is not "anti-medicine" or "anti-surgery," although I will say emphatically that chiropractic remains "anti-unnecessary surgery" and "anti-unnecessary medications." Most of all, chiropractic remains steadfastly for freedom of choice in health care, a principle that political medicine has long resisted in our country. Let's give the public the best of both worlds in health care.

If you believe there must be a better way to get well than relying upon drugs and surgery, hopefully the abundance of research from around the world will help convince you to seek a chiropractor before you consider back surgery. The evidence is clear that spinal manipulation is the best initial form of treatment for the vast majority of back problems and the research also demonstrates the gross ineffectiveness of back surgery. The ultimate decision about your spinal problem must come from an informed understanding of the benefits of chiropractic care. That understanding only occurs when you begin to think out of the "medical box" of solutions.

A good example of the change in attitude many informed people make once they understand chiropractic and forget the propaganda of the medical misinformants is the consensus of the New Zealand Commission of Inquiry. This study into chiropractic, conducted from 1978-79, was the most thorough governmental investigation at the time:

"We entered into our inquiry in early 1978. We had no clear idea what might emerge. We knew little about chiropractors. None of us had undergone any personal experience of chiropractic treatment. If we had any general impression of chiropractic, it was probably that shared by many in the community: that chiropractic was an unscientific cult, not to be compared with orthodox medical or paramedical services. We might well have thought that chiropractors were people with perhaps a strong urge for healing, who had for some reason not been able to get into a field recognized by orthodox medicine and who had found an outlet outside the fringes of orthodoxy.

"But as we prepared ourselves for this inquiry it became apparent that much lay beneath the surface of these apparently simple terms of reference. In the first place, it transpired that for many years chiropractors had been making strenuous efforts to gain recognition and acceptance as members of the established health-care team. Secondly, it was clear that organized medicine in New Zealand was adamantly opposed to this on a variety of grounds which appeared logical and responsible. Thirdly, however, it became only too plain that the argument had been going on ever since chiropractic was developed as an individual discipline in the late 1800s, and that in the years between then and now the debate had generated considerably more heat than light.

"By the end of the inquiry we found ourselves irresistibly and with complete unanimity drawn to the conclusion that modern chiropractic is a soundly-based and valuable branch of health-care in a specialized area... For the vast majority of neck and back pain sufferers, however, chiropractic offers a conservative alternative which studies show may yield effective, quick relief from pain."[15]

Just as this commission's initial opinion was changed from skepticism to an informed, positive judgment by investigation of the facts about chiropractic, the same transformation occurs every day in every chiropractic clinic when patients finally learn the truth about this great science. The most common statement I hear from these converts is, "It's so logical." It also comes as a shock for many patients to realize they have been lied to by their MD about chiropractic care. After years of suffering with back pain, living on useless pain pills or, even worse, undergoing back surgery that failed, many patients ask me, "Why didn't my MD tell me to go to a chiropractor first?" Indeed, once you understand chiropractic and not just believe the medical hearsay and misinformation, you too will think the same.

Actually, the public's opinion of chiropractic is changing despite the medical resistance. In 1989, D.C. Cherkin, MD, and F.A. MacCornack, MD, researched patient evaluation of low back pain care from family physicians and chiropractors and chiropractic patients were found to be "three times as likely as patients of family physicians to report that they were very satisfied with the care they received for low back pain (66 percent vs. 22 percent, respectively).[16]

A Gallup Organization poll reported in March 1991 examined the attitudes and behaviors of both users and non-users of chiropractic services. Of the chiropractic patients, 90 percent felt chiropractic treatment was effective; more than 80 percent were satisfied with their treatment; nearly 75 percent felt most of their expectations had been met during their visits; 68 percent said they would see a chiropractor again for treatment of a similar condition; and 50 percent would likely see a chiropractor again for other conditions. Of the non-users of chiropractic services, 62 percent responded they would see a doctor of chiropractic for a problem applicable to chiropractic treatment; 25 percent reported that someone in their household had been treated by a chiropractor and nearly 80 percent of those were satisfied with the chiropractic treatment received.[17]

Although millions of people now utilize alternative health care, many still are unaware of the new revelations about its effectiveness. For the most part, the media gives only a small notice to these revolutionary findings, and it just as quickly escapes from the public consciousness. Moreover, patients remain uninformed about this new spinal research when their local MD downplays the importance of these new findings and continues to prescribe pills and surgery instead of referring patients to a chiropractor. In fact, it remains difficult for the average patient to gain access to the best solution to this epidemic of back problems despite the newest scientific research and governmental endorsements. This is because the mainstream medical world is very slow to change its ineffective methods or to refer to a chiropractor, especially if it doesn't profit! In fact, it's ultimately up to you to find the truth about this pervasive problem of back pain because the medical world rarely tells the whole truth about chiropractic care. Consumer beware!

Sound Too Familiar?

As you read this book, keep in mind the experiences of just a few of the many patients, perhaps people just like yourself, who have been helped by chiropractic care after years of failed medical care.

Diane is a 39-year-old woman who had been disabled by low back pain for 15 years. Her Workers' Compensation doctors had filled her with pills and performed extensive physical therapy and diagnostic exams, all to no avail. She was scheduled to undergo exploratory back surgery, although the MRI test could not find any reason for it – no ruptured or degenerated discs, no bone spurs or factures or pathologies of any sort. Diane simply had unrelenting, intense back pain after her on-the-job accident. When she asked her MD if she could consult a chiropractor before surgery, he adamantly denied her request and told her, "Chiropractors will only make you worse!"

Nevertheless, with great trepidation, Diane came to my office seeking help. Years before her accident her husband had used chiropractic care successfully, and Diane said she was afraid of back surgery. After only three spinal adjustments, by her own admission Diane was 75 percent pain-free. In reality, hers was an easy case, since she only needed her spinal joints adjusted. Yet her MD had misdiagnosed her, mistreated her, failed to give her informed consent about options to his care and failed to refer her for the correct type of care – chiropractic. Her case had cost her insurance company thousands of wasted dollars and more importantly, had cost her 15 of the best years of her life.

> **The solution is to think out of the medical box!**
> Chiropractic
>
> Exercise   Medical Box   Weight Loss
> Drugs
> Hospitalizations
> Surgeries
>
> Posture
>
> **Without lifting your pencil, connect the 9 dots using only 4 straight lines.**

Colonel K. is an Air Force officer who had four back surgeries and was scheduled to undergo a fifth. A junior officer, a patient of mine, brought him into my office for a consultation. The colonel, a medically-tainted skeptic, informed me of his disbelief in chiropractic: "If my saintly neurosurgeon can't help me with four surgeries, how can you? Why, you can't even give me drugs!" So, I asked the colonel if he had ever played poker, because there's an old adage that says, "You shouldn't throw good money in after bad." Apparently he never had heard of this principle.

After only two weeks of chiropractic care, the colonel was angry. When I asked him why, he said, "I'm 88 percent pain-free. Why didn't my surgeon send me to a chiropractor first?"

"Good question," I responded. "The next time you see him, why don't you ask him that very question. And when he tells you that chiropractic care doesn't work, and now you know it does, then you'll know he can't be trusted with your health." The colonel, like many failed back surgery victims, had every right to be angry – it's no fun having four back surgeries, especially when they are unnecessary and ineffective.

Teresa's migraines started 25 years before I met her. When she was only five years old she was involved in a car accident and hit her head on the windshield because she wasn't wearing a seat belt. Since then she has spent over $125,000 for specialists, hospitals, tests, and of course, endless strong prescription drugs, all to no avail, because she still experienced daily migraine headaches. I met Teresa at a Migraine Sufferers' Society meeting when I spoke about the chiropractic solution to migraine headaches – adjusting the top vertebrae in the spine.

Shortly thereafter Teresa reluctantly came to see me as her proverbial "last resort" and announced to me that she was skeptical of chiropractors. Knowing of her failed medical care, I asked if she was skeptical of medical doctors after spending 25 years and over $125,000 on their failed care? She got my point that perhaps her skepticism was misplaced, inasmuch as she had never before had chiropractic care.

Within two weeks of receiving neck adjustments, Teresa's migraines were gone. After only a few adjustments, I entered the treatment room one day and she was crying. I asked her if her headaches were back and she said that they weren't, and that was exactly why she was crying – out of joy and relief. She said, "Do you know what it's like to have a migraine for 25 years? My tears are from my happiness not to wake up with a migraine. Thank you so much."

I simply replied, "Don't thank me, thank chiropractic care."

Mrs. T. had five back surgeries within just a few years. She still had as much pain after the last surgery as she did before the first. When she asked her surgeon why she still hurt, he told her, "I don't know. I got all the disc."

When she told me this story, I simply responded to her, "Mrs. T., did you ever think your pain may not be coming from your discs? Perhaps it's coming from your spinal joints."

"Oh," she replied in disbelief. "He never mentioned that possibility." MDs rarely do tell their patients the whole truth about their pain and their treatment options.

Do any of these true accounts sound painfully familiar to you? These are but a few examples of the millions of people who were medical failures but who have had great results from chiropractic care. Despite their initial skepticism and medical prejudice, the good results they achieved with chiropractic care not only helped their headaches and back pain, but opened up their minds to another world of health-care. They found, as you will too, that chiropractic care is good for much more than back pain. Indeed, you don't need just a backache to see a chiropractor!

If you're like Diane, Colonel K., Teresa or Mrs. T., I urge you to seek care from a professional doctor of chiropractic. Unfortunately, too many people fall victim to unnecessary back surgery and dangerous, ineffective drugs that, by and large, do little good. Don't use chiropractic care as the "last resort" as many patients do and don't be mislead or discouraged because your MD, family or friends are medically-tainted and may be ignorant about the benefits which chiropractic offers. Every year thousands upon thousands of patients suffer from failed back surgeries that are mostly preventable. And every year millions upon millions of people discover chiropractic care and use it as a "first resort" to their back problems.

Unfortunately, too many patients fall prey to medical misinformation about back problems. For example, Paulette came to my office and couldn't even sit or stand for more than a few minutes because of intense low back pain – I actually consulted with her while she was lying down! She had been disabled for five weeks, living on pain pills and muscle relaxants, and was told she had two herniated discs that needed surgery. Her husband and a co-worker urged her to come to my office instead, but it became obvious to me this woman didn't want my help. After a lengthy discussion about her condition and the new guideline that suggests conservative care before any surgery, she still was quite skeptical. She asked, "Why didn't the surgeon recommend chiropractic?" I told her that would be equivalent of a Republican referring a voter to a Democrat and isn't likely to happen when there's a $25,000 surgical fee involved.

Despite the facts, Paulette decided not to give chiropractic care a chance, and elected to have back surgery. Apparently her MD had given her the *voo-doo* diagnosis: "If you don't have my surgery, you'll get worse. And if you go to a chiropractor, he'll paralyze you." Sadly, too many "Paulettes" have listened to the wrong advice, chosen the path of drugs and surgery, only to suffer for the rest of their lives. Don't make this same mistake yourself!

Medical Gall

Much of the dilemma about back pain care rests with the fact that most MDs are not spinal specialists, although they might appear to be. In fact, as you will learn, most MDs know practically nothing about this most important part of your body. For example, ask your MD how many joints are in the spinal column and watch him or her choke with embarrassment!

Unfortunately, medical incompetency in the area of musculoskeletal problems has long been a problem within the professional ranks, although it is unknown to the public. Some people mistakenly think their local MD actually is an expert on the spine. It never ceases to amaze me the incorrect diagnoses from MDs that are brought to my office by their disgruntled failed medical patients.

For example – and there are many to chose from – a young female attorney came to see me with chronic low back pain. Her family MD told her she had a simple "pulled muscle" syndrome that would go away with muscle relaxants.

"That was five years ago," she said. She asked me expectantly, "Shouldn't it be gone by now?"

After my chiropractic spinal analysis, I found her low back pain was a combination of problems, none of which was a "pulled" muscle. She had a short leg syndrome causing a very titled pelvis, sacralization of her lumbar spine, decompensatory lumbar scoliosis, she was slightly overweight and was in a very deconditioned state with weak abdominal and back muscles. In fact, this woman had many spinal problems, none of which was a "pulled" muscle. Too often, patients are misdiagnosed by incompetent MDs who try to be experts on everything to everybody, and their simplistic spinal diagnoses always end up to be the proverbial "pulled muscle" or "slipped disc" or, if that fails, then the advice, "It's all in your head."

It is a little known fact that the average MD knows precious little about back pain. Too many patients fail to realize that most MDs have never studied the science or art of spinal care. As far back as November 1966, an article titled, "Manipulation for Backache and Sciatica," appeared in the *Journal of Applied Therapeutics* by W.B. Parsons, MD, and H.K. Boake, MD, who wrote about this dilemma:

> "Yet how many physicians know anything of this method of treatment [chiropractic] that can help a high percentage of their patients? <u>These things are not taught in medical schools. Usually the concept is condemned so that new doctors go out in the world with no knowledge, or even worse, an antipathy toward this most useful method.</u> Their pills, potions, and applications do little good. Even if the nature of the origin of the complaint is recognized and the patient is sent for standard physiotherapy, usually little relief is obtained. Often the patient then goes to another office [chiropractic], his spine is mobilized [adjusted], his symptom relieved and the doctor has lost a case."[18]

One interesting note about the lack of medical training in this area was revealed unexpectedly during the chiropractic vs. AMA anti-trust trial (*Wilk* case) in Chicago which ended in 1987 after nearly 12 years of hearings, trials and appeals all the way to the U.S. Supreme Court, which let the lower court's decision stand in favor of the chiropractic plaintiffs. The Supreme Court declined to review a Trial Court and Court of Appeals finding that the AMA had been guilty of a "lengthy, systematic, successful, and unlawful boycott" of doctors of chiropractic and their patients.

U.S. district court Judge Susan Getzendanner handed down a judgement against the AMA, the American College of Surgeons and the American College of Radiology, stating they did conspire to destroy the chiropractic profession. This landmark legal decision denounced the "lawlessness" and years of "objectively unreasonable" persecution and bigotry by the AMA's political goons. The judge also discovered much more than just a conspiracy; she found that many general practitioners actually were posing as experts in this realm of health care, and that chiropractors were more qualified in these cases.

"But, according to the Court (and this is unchallenged), at the same time, there was evidence before the committee that chiropractic was effective, indeed more effective than the medical profession, in treating certain kinds of problems, such as back injuries. The committee was also aware, the Court found, that some medical physicians believed chiropractic could be effective and that chiropractors were better trained to deal with musculoskeletal problems than most medical physicians."[19]

At one point during this federal court trial, a renowned orthopedic surgeon, John McMillan Mennell, MD, who has taught in many medical schools, testified that the average MD has approximately four classroom hours on the musculoskeletal system, which comprises over 60 percent of the human body, and no classroom training on spinal manipulation.[20] That's equivalent of one class to cover the majority of the human body! The judge was astounded to realize how little the MDs actually knew about the musculoskeletal system or manipulation, inasmuch as they appeared to the average patient to be all-knowing experts.

In fact, in 1988 researchers Drs. Cherkin and MacCornack surveyed MDs and DCs in Washington state to determine their beliefs and attitudes about low back pain (LBP). Their findings were stunning in that "42% of family physicians felt they had been poorly trained to manage low back pain." Other findings were just as shocking: Most MDs (47%) believe "muscle strain" was the major reason and were more likely to think the causes to be psychosomatic ("It's all in your head"). Many MDs (88%) also believed LBP would resolve itself within a few weeks; only 31% believed that a precise diagnosis was necessary; 19% actually felt there was nothing wrong with many patients who complain of LBP; and only 2% of MDs thought LBP was due to joint dysfunction or vertebral subluxation. Due to their inadequate training about musculoskeletal problems, faulty assumptions about the causes of LBP (disc abnormalities/muscle strain), combined with ineffective treatments (pills/surgery) explain why only 55% of MDs who felt that most of their patients were satisfied with the care they rendered.[21]

It's frightening to realize how little MDs know about this epidemic of back pain. What they are taught about back pain is that the problem is either a "pulled muscle" or "slipped disc." And their treatment consists of pain pills and muscle relaxants, and when that fails, disc surgery is the next and only recommendation. They rarely mention the likelihood of joint dysfunction as the cause of back pain, nor are they taught to refer to chiropractors. And we wonder why patients are mismanaged, when their family doctor is filled with prejudice, poorly trained and works from faulty information about America's number one health problem?

On the other hand, researchers have found that chiropractic patients were highly satisfied with their care. Again, Drs. Cherkin and MacCornack compared patient satisfaction with chiropractic and physician management of LBP and concluded that "the percentage of chiropractic patients who were 'very satisfied' with the care they received for low back pain was triple that for patients of family physicians."[22] Undoubtedly, patients are impressed by more thorough exams, better explanations of their problem and more effective treatment plans. This research verified that the reason the public has long supported chiropractors was because their methods were more clinically and cost-effective than medical methods.

It must take quite a bit of gall for medical professionals to bash chiropractors, when in fact, they have no idea what we do or how we do it. Further, they know that chiropractors are better at diagnosing and treating most back pain cases, anyway. They just refuse to tell their patients the truth, and considering the plethora of research and the new guideline endorsing chiropractic care, their antagonism can only be based on historical prejudice or market share competition. It may also be simply the result of believing their own lies and delusions for years that has led many medical professionals to an irrational condemnation of chiropractors.

We wonder why our nation has an epidemic of back pain. With insurance companies restricting chiropractic care, precious little available through the press to the public about the best solution, combined with antagonistic MDs who refuse to refer cases to DCs, you have the makings of a disaster, which is just what has happened. Forget about which treatments work best and least costly; forget about what the research supports and the federal government endorses; and forget about what patients want. Political medicine has no interest in your well-being unless it can exclusively profit.

P. Joseph Lisa mentioned this medical malpractice and patient predicament: "Consumers: Do not wait for some doctor to tell you, 'Your mother is dead. We did all we could do to save her. There was nothing more we could do. She had the best treatment medicine could give her. Sorry!' <u>That is the Big Lie. They didn't do everything they could have done, because they never gave you or her a chance to find out if an alternative treatment could save her life. There was something more that they could do, but they wouldn't dare send you to their competition. They have too many dollars to lose.</u> They didn't give her the 'best treatment medicine could offer.' Other treatments out there that are much less expensive might have saved her life. They would never tell you about them."[23]

Every day millions of Americans with back pain are being told the Big Lie about chiropractic and are railroaded into expensive and ineffective medical management by myopic MDs and discriminatory insurance policies which deny or restrict chiropractic care. The consequences are staggeringly expensive – $100 billion annually on direct and indirect costs – and in terms of human suffering, the loss is incalculable. Even now, when the U.S. Public Health Service guideline on acute low back pain is well known, the medical profession continues to ignore it because of their potential loss of profit. The epidemic of back attacks that Americans face is not a matter of coincidence or merely bad luck. It has been the design of the AMA to profit from this epidemic by suppressing a viable alternative that has proven to be more effective and less costly than the medical mismanagement of drugs and back surgeries. There's just too much money to lose for the surgeons and the hospitals which average $14,000 for one disc surgery. Of course, it rarely ends at just one surgery, because many failed back surgery patients undergo more than one. Indeed, there's too much money at stake to let the chiropractic solution stand in their way.

Blind Faith and Skepticism

Before anyone can be convinced that the best solution to most all back pain is chiropractic care, it's important to start with an open mind and a clean slate about this problem. For too long the chiropractic profession has taken a huge public relations beating from the medical profession which has confused the public through the media with scary stories – most often embellishments of rare, accidental occurrences. Few people have a clear picture of chiropractic, and many don't get that picture until they enter a chiropractor's office. If you've been tainted by medical misinformation about chiropractic care, as many people have been, I urge you to keep an open mind on this subject because you may be shocked as you learn the truth about the epidemic of back attacks. Many patients have learned after receiving chiropractic care that it's no fun to realize they've been mislead about the best form of care for their back pain, especially after they've had a failed back surgery. This happens more often than most people realize. When the U.S. Public Health Service report on acute low back pain says that only one in 100 back surgeries is helpful, something is obviously wrong.

Another co-factor in this epidemic of back pain has been the public's "blind faith" in medicine. Its willingness to accept without question any and all medical decisions has lead to massive drug abuse (such as we're now experiencing with "super-germ" infections from the overuse of antibiotics), and many unnecessary surgical procedures like back surgery, hysterectomies, tonsillectomies and coronary bypass surgeries, to name but a few of the many unnecessary surgical scams performed routinely in our country. When medical experts like Lynn Payer writes in her book, *Disease-Mongers*, that 78 percent to 90 percent of all surgeries are deemed unnecessary, something is amiss.[24] Much of this fact can be attributed to unsuspecting, naive patients who simply do as they are told or do as they are scared into doing so by a *voo-doo* medical diagnosis.

Patients' unquestioning belief in their MDs' decisions also often includes subscribing to the medical bigotry against chiropractic. Rather than making an informed decision based on facts, too many people merely follow the biased recommendations of their medics for a variety of reasons. Some MDs would refuse to see patients if they did use chiropractors; some MDs would disseminate untruths about chiropractic care; and some MDs would ridicule patients even for asking about alternatives to drugs and surgery. For many patients, it becomes a symbol of their loyalty to their MDs to buy into the bigotry and to naively bash chiropractic. Unfortunately for them, their "blind faith" loyalty ends up in many failed back surgeries that could easily have been prevented with chiropractic care. And this bigotry has fueled the fire of misinformation that has added greatly to the cost and tragedy of this epidemic of back pain.

It's quite normal to have a healthy skepticism about new ideas, especially those that are different from the status quo. I understand that most people have no real understanding about chiropractic spinal care and how adjustments can solve their back pain. And I certainly understand that even fewer people comprehend how chiropractic may help organic problems by correcting nerve pressure. After consulting with thousands of average people, I have come to expect them to be filled with fears, worries and concerns due to their own lack of understanding and the years of medical misinformation. Long before I examine them and begin a treatment program, I make it a point to inquire about whatever emotional feelings about chiropractic they may have. I do so to resolve these misunderstandings upfront so they don't interfere with the treatment program later on. Sometimes dealing with this skepticism is the largest problem I encounter in the healing process. However, I certainly don't want patients simply to *believe in* chiropractic through blind faith. I prefer that they *understand* the logic and science of our care so they get the best results possible. Chiropractic is a science, not a religion, and the more you learn about this natural health-care science, the more you will learn about how to avoid back surgery and the holistic health benefits chiropractic care offers.

Much of the misinformation about the cause and correction of spinal problems continues today despite the overwhelming deluge of scientific research and government endorsements over the last few years. Whether it's disc surgery, rods implanted in the spine, spinal fusions, laminectomies, or pedicle screws in the spine, for the most part these medical methods have proven ineffective, very expensive, and in many cases, permanently disabling. Despite the scientific research which supports spinal manipulation as the most effective form of spinal care, to this day, if you were to poll the average American about what causes back pain, most people would say "pulled muscles" or "slipped discs." And if you were to ask them what the best solutions are, again they most likely would say, "pain pills, muscles relaxants and back surgery." If you want to avoid back surgery, and 99 percent are avoidable, the first thing you must do is to forget what the medical misinformation has taught you.

I say it's time to douse the fire of bigotry, no matter from what source it may arise – especially from the MDs atop their pedestals. As you learn about this dilemma of back pain, you will see how chiropractors have withstood these flames of prejudice and, like the proverbial phoenix, have risen from over a century of discrimination to stand vindicated today with the realization that chiropractic has been on the right path all along. For the weary DCs who have fought this bigotry for decades, the real fruits of their battle rest with the greater opportunity today to share with everyone the benefits of chiropractic care and to help more people avoid back surgery and a life of disability.

This book is intended for those patients seeking a non-surgical, drugless and highly effective solution to their back pain. The key to solving your back pain and avoiding back surgery begins with a new perspective about this 20th century disaster. The answer exists to solving this number one epidemic striking Americans, but the solution lies outside the mainstream of medical drugs and surgical methods. I suggest you learn to think out of the "medical box" if your goal is to avoid back surgery – the huge costs, possible disability and the frustration of ineffective surgical outcomes. In fact, your ability to think out the box of medical solutions will be the catalyst in a transformation process that may be one of the biggest attitudinal changes in your life. And it is one that is essential if your goal is to avoid back surgery. The paradigm shift from the medical box to the chiropractic model is no less of a change than changing political parties or churches. As your awareness about health care evolves, you will naturally change many of your attitudes and opinions. I only hope you discover the benefits of chiropractic spinal care before you or someone you know falls victim to the epidemic of failed back surgery in America.

U.S. Public Health Service Guidelines For Acute Low Back Pain

EXCERPTS FROM PATIENT GUIDE

Proven Treatments

Spinal Manipulation

This treatment (using the hands to apply force to the back to "adjust" the spine) can be helpful for some people in the first month of low back symptoms. **It should only be done by a professional with experience in manipulation.**

Heat or cold applied to the back. Within the first 48 hours after your back symptoms start, you may want to apply a cold pack (or a bag of ice) to the painful area for 5 to 10 minutes at a time.

Medicine often helps relieve low back symptoms. The type of medicine that your health care provider recommends depends on your symptoms and how uncomfortable you are.

If your symptoms are mild to moderate, you may get the relief you need from an over-the-counter (non-prescription) medicine such as acetaminophen, aspirin, or ibuprofen. These medicines ususally have fewer side effects than prescription medicines and are less expensive.

If your symptoms are severe, your health care provider may recommend a prescription medicine.

Other Treatments

A number of other treatments are sometimes used for low back symptoms. While these treatments may give relief for a short time, none have been found to speed recovery or keep acute back problems from returning. They may also be expensive. Such treatments include:

Traction
TENS (transcutaneous electrical nerve stimulation)
Massage
Biofeedback
Acupuncture
Injections into the back
Back Corsets
Ultrasound

About Surgery

Even having a lot of back pain does not by itself mean you need surgery. **Surgery has been found to be helpful in only 1 in 100 cases of low back problems.** In some people, surgery can even cause more problems. This is especially true if your only symptom is back pain.

People with certain nerve problems or conditions such as fractures or dislocations have the best chance of being helped by surgery. In most cases however, decisions about surgery do not have to be made right away. Most back surgery can wait for several weeks without making the condition worse.

If your health care provider recommends surgery, be sure to ask about the reason for the surgery and about the risks and benefits you might expect. You may also want to get a second opinion.

Referenced from the Agency for Health Care Policy and Research, 1994, "Acute Low Back Pain in Adults"

CHAPTER THREE

The Epidemic of Back Surgery

"Traditional medical treatment has failed to halt this epidemic and may even have contributed to it. There is a clear need to reconsider our whole approach to the management of low back pain and disability."
– Her Majesty's Stationery Office in London in its *Report of a Clinical Standards Advisory Group Committee on Back Pain,* 1994.

ack pain in America is an epidemic that has been virtually ignored for decades, mismanaged badly by the medical profession and has now become a very expensive problem that will affect 80 percent of all adults sometime in their lifetime. Consider these facts from a 1994 report from the U.S. Public Health Service on Acute Low Back Pain in Adults[1]:

1. National statistics indicate a yearly prevalence rate of 15-20 percent.
2. Among work-age people, 50 percent admit to experiencing back symptoms.
3. Back symptoms are the most common cause of disability for persons under the age of 45.
4. At any given time, about 1 percent of the U.S. population is chronically disabled because of back symptoms, and another 1 percent is temporarily disabled.
5. Low back problems (LBPs) are the second most common reason for office visits to primary care physicians.
6. LBP ranks third among the reasons for undergoing surgical procedures.
7. Estimates of total annual cost of back pain in the U.S. range from $20 to $75 billion.
8. About 2 percent of the U.S. work force reports compensable back problems each year.
9. There is increasing evidence that many patients may be receiving care that is inappropriate or at least less than optimal.
10. Some patients appear to be more disabled after treatment than before, another potential indicator of suboptimal care – the most obvious examples involve surgery.

This most startling study on low back pain management was released in December 1994 by the U.S. Department of Health and Human Services. Its own Public Health Service created the Agency for Health Care Policy and Research (AHCPR), by request of the U.S. Congress in 1989, to investigate important health problems in our country. Their mission was to conduct research into "medical effectiveness research, facilitating development of clinical practice guidelines, and disseminating research findings and guidelines to health-care providers, policy-makers and to the public."

The AHCPR convened a 23-member panel of medical and chiropractic doctors, nurses, experts in spine research, physical therapists, psychologists and occupational therapists. Its guideline is based on a review of all the existing medical literature on the treatment of low back pain – over 4,000 articles from the Library of Congress. This expert panel, chaired by Stanley Bigos, MD, orthopedic surgeon, in its "Clinical Practice Guideline" for practitioners, stated emphatically:

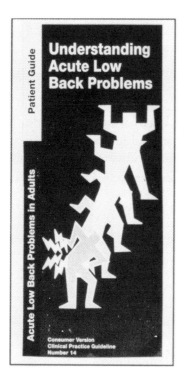

"Despite an extensive medical literature on 'failed back surgery' and evidence that repeat surgical procedures for low back problems rarely lead to improved outcome, there are documented examples of patients who have had as many as 20 spine operations. However, surgery is not the only treatment that can lead to increased disability. Common treatment methods such as extended bed rest or extended use of high-dose opioids can prolong symptoms and further debilitate patients."[2]

The AHCPR concluded that spinal manipulation is the best initial form of professional treatment for the vast majority of back pain cases, and that back surgery is mostly unnecessary. *"Surgery helps only one in 100 people with acute low back problems,"* according to the AHCPR guideline. The guideline also states quite clearly that *"Even having a lot of back pain does not by itself mean you need surgery."* [3]

It's one thing for Britain or Canada or Workers' Compensation studies to criticize back surgery and recommend chiropractic care, but when a U.S. government panel of medical experts does so, red flags should go up to the public that the medical management is currently on the wrong track. It should also be a warning to consumers that despite the new guideline from the U.S. Public Health Service, much of the medical profession still ignores the new recommendations. The intransigence of the AMA to the new guideline on acute low back pain typifies their constant pattern to ignore research that criticizes their methods and would decrease their profiteering. Indeed, consumer beware!

Not only did the AHCPR rate spinal manipulation highest on the list of effective treatments for acute low back pain, it also rated the standard medical procedures such as surgery, injections of anesthetics and corticosteroids very low. Also criticized were the methods used by physical therapists – ultrasound, traction, TENS, massage – all of which are expensive and which provide short-term relief at best. Every comparison of clinical results has shown that spinal manipulation is clearly superior to standard physical therapy methods which were found to give only temporary results, and that it is superior to expensive back surgeries which were found in many cases to be unnecessary and disabling.

After years of research, many medical and independent experts agree that the medical management of back pain with bed rest, pain pills, muscle relaxants and back surgery just hasn't proven to be either clinical or cost-effective. When you consider that 70 percent of neurosurgeons' incomes come from operations on the spine -- spinal fusions, pedicle screws, laminectomies and discectomies – if the new guideline helps patients to avoid these radical surgeries, it will put quite a dent in health-care costs.

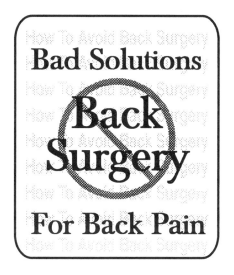

At the December 8, 1994 press conference introducing the guideline on acute low back pain in adults, Philip R. Lee, MD, assistant secretary for Health and Human Services and head of the Public Health Services said: "These guidelines could save Americans considerable anguish, time and much money now spent on unneeded or unproved medical care." I find it interesting that Dr. Lee did not say, "unproven chiropractic care" – he specifically said "medical" care. Clifton R. Gaus, Sc.D., administrator of AHCPR, also mentioned in the news release that, "... a preliminary cost analysis of these guidelines suggests the nation could save as much as a third of the medical expense of treating this condition without any loss of quality of care."

Actually, after years of criticism and calls for research and proof about chiropractic care, I think the AMA now wishes the issue had been left alone and unnoticed, since the new evidence proves what surgeons were doing was ineffective, risky and expensive, and that chiropractors were right all along!

In 1993 the Manga Report from the Ontario Ministry of Health titled, "The Effectiveness and Cost-Effectiveness of Chiropractic Management of Low-Back Pain," made an equally strong impact by concluding that spinal manipulation was best form of care.

> "There is overwhelming body of evidence indicating that chiropractic management of low-back pain is more cost-effective than medical management. We reviewed numerous studies that range from very persuasive to convincing in support of this conclusion. The lack of any convincing argument or evidence to the contrary must be noted and is significant to us in forming our conclusions and recommendations. The evidence includes studies showing lower chiropractic costs for the same diagnosis and episodic

need for care. There should be highly significant cost savings if more management of LBP (low back pain) was transferred from physicians to chiropractors."[4]

The British Research Council (Meade Report) conducted an extensive ten-year study which compared chiropractic and medical management of low back pain. It was reported in the *British Medical Journal* in 1990 and came to the same conclusion, that chiropractic care is the most clinical and cost-effective form of treatment for low back pain. "The potential economic, resource and policy implications of our results are extensive." The council's conclusions were that chiropractic treatment is significantly more effective, particularly for patients with chronic and severe pain. Results were long-term – "the benefits of chiropractic treatment became more evident throughout the follow-up period of two years." It urged that "Consideration should be given...to providing chiropractic within the NHS (National Health Services) either in hospitals or by purchasing chiropractic treatment from existing clinics." The council's economic analysis shows savings in excess of ten million British pounds per annum by treating hospitals' outpatients with back pain with chiropractors.[5]

Despite the growing evidence against back surgeries, there has been a dramatic increase in their number since 1980, primarily due to the complete lack of guidelines, unquestioned insurance coverage and professional profiteering. Data from a national survey indicated that between 1980 and 1990, spinal surgeries increased 137 percent, while the population older than 25 rose only by 23 percent. One researcher, Dr. Casey Lee noted that the surgery rates were in direct proportion to the ratio of surgeons to populations. For example, between 1980 and 1990, the number of neurosurgeons and orthopedic surgeons increased by 24 percent. In his speech, "Challenges of the Spine Specialists," Dr. Lee, 1993-'94 president of the North American Spine Society, stated:

"The number of operations for spinal disorders, especially disc excision and spinal fusion, have been steadily rising over the years; 75 percent and 200 percent change from 1979 to 1987, respectively, for discectomy and spinal fusion.

"...the rate of laminectomy for disc herniation in the United States is three times higher than in Canada and nine times higher than in Europe... The rate of spinal fusion in the western region of United States is nine times higher than in the Northeast.

"Reasons for these variations are lack of uniquely successful diagnostic and therapeutic approaches and lack of consensus in diagnosis and management. This implies that there is very little scientific basis for clinical practice, and the conventional method for care is wasteful and pernicious."[6]

Another study, conducted in 1994 by Drs. D.C. Cherkin, R.A. Deyo, J.D. Loeser, T. Bush, and G. Waddell comparing international rates of back surgeries revealed the startling fact that American surgeons are unusually excessive: "The rate of back surgery in the United States was at least 40 percent higher than any other country and was more than five times those in England and Scotland. Back surgery rates increased almost linearly with the per capita supply of orthopedic and neurosurgeons in the country."[7]

According to another study conducted by H. Davis, MD, which appeared in *Spine* magazine revealed that the surgery rates between 1980 and 1990 were increasing in a shocking manner:

> "[T]he rate of hospitalization with cervical spine surgery increased more than 45 percent with the rates for cervical fusion surgery increasing more than 70 percent. The rate of hospitalization with lumbar spine surgery increased more than 33 percent in each sex, with the rate of lumbar fusion surgery increasing more than 60 percent in each sex, the rate for lumbar disc surgery increasing more than 40 percent among males and 21 percent among females, and the rate for lumbar exploration/ decompression surgery increasing more than 65 percent in each sex."[8]

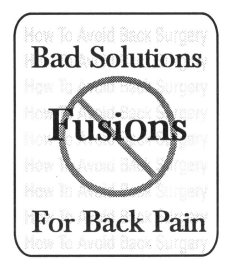

In fact, this misadventure of spinal surgery not only has been mostly ineffective, it is a worse-case scenario of professional intransigence founded on a false premise that has left thousands of patients disabled. It is a sensitive issue about which many ethical medical professionals have long warned their colleagues. "The surgeon who believes that his scalpel can cure the ills of the cervical spine should take time to live with his patients before and after surgery. If he does this, he would be more cautious in the selection of patients for cervical surgery... The patient's future must be of prime concern." [9]

While this admonition sounds like it comes from a chiropractor, in fact, it came from one of the leading medical experts in the field of orthopedic surgery, Ruth Jackson, MD, FACS. The medical literature itself is replete with caution and criticism for back surgery, although it seems to have fallen on deaf ears. Dr. Ruth Jackson, formerly chief of orthopedic surgery at Parkland Hospital and an instructor at Baylor University College of Medicine in Dallas, wrote the mainstay of medical textbooks on neck problems, titled *The Cervical Syndrome*. The first edition was published as long ago as 1956.

> "Surgery should be avoided unless there are absolute and definite indications for it, otherwise the results from operative procedures will be disappointing and the symptoms may be worse than they were before surgery.
>
> "... <u>Fusion of two or more vertebrae places a greater strain on the adjacent movable vertebral joints to give rise to continued symptoms and the necessity, apparently, for further fusions.</u>
>
> "...Arthur Steindler, MD, has stated that patience as well as study are required in the treatment of the complex cervical spine disorders. The

deplorable trend to short-circuit these responsibilities by precipitate operations, the disdaining of conservative efforts as useless wastes of time and the uncompromising attitude of generalizing operative indications has done nothing to establish a wholesome equilibrium between radical action and conservative expectation, but, on the contrary, has contributed much to cloud the issue.

"...Steindler often said 'There are those who wish to go non-stop, and in their haste pass by the stations of indications and diagnosis, to arrive at specific operative techniques. No doubt they will be disappointed.' There has been a rash of surgical procedures for cervical spine disorders during the past two decades. How many operations should really have been done we will never, in all probability, know."[10]

Not just rogue surgeons are to blame for the startling increase in back surgeries; the insurance industry must shoulder some of the blame as well. While insurance companies complain about the rising costs of medical care, many nonetheless still exclude chiropractic care from coverage, despite the overwhelming evidence that most back pain responds best to manipulative therapy. This obvious duplicity is due to the fact that too many MDs sit on the board of directors of most insurance companies. Not only have their decisions denied patients the freedom to select a more effective, non-invasive method to solve their back attacks, they actually have railroaded patients into ineffective, costly, and mostly unnecessary back surgeries.

In those states where HMOs attempt to contain costs, back surgeries were found to be "roughly half the rates for the states in which the HMOs were located and where fee-for-service practice and easy access to surgeons is the norm." The study by Drs. Cherkin and Deyo suggested that differences in "financial incentives to perform surgery and in practice style philosophies" may explain why HMO back surgery rates are much lower. I dare add that if all HMOs included chiropractors, these rates would be even lower. Drs. Cherkin and Deyo estimate that approximately $1 billion per year is wasted on hospitalization of patients with low back pain. They estimate that up to 70 percent of hospitalization and 80 percent of hospital days for back pain problems are inappropriate and unnecessary. In Washington state, after stricter guidelines were instituted, Drs. Cherkin and Deyo noted a decrease of 47 percent in hospitalization for low back pain patients.[11]

The rash of unnecessary back surgery is not a new issue, although it is escalating. In their article titled, "An Historical Perspective on Low-Back Pain and Disability," authors David B. Allan, MD and Dr. Gordon Waddell mentions that low back pain is not a new problem and the disability rate is actually enhanced by medical methods.

"Backache has affected human beings throughout reported history... This growth in disability is closely related to medical management of backache... Sadly, we must conclude that much low-back disability is iatrogenic [doctor-caused]."[12]

Their criticism focused on medical over-reaction to disc problems with the advent of x-ray, when two early orthopedic surgeons, Drs. Mixter and Barr's 1934 paper shifted the attention of sciatica to the intervertebral disc:

> "These moves away from the early strict criteria unleashed on the unsuspecting public a wave of surgical enthusiasm hindered only by World War II. The concept of 'disc lesions' was constantly extended to explain backache quite illogically and unjustifiably, particularly by orthopedic surgeons who were keen to re-establish their role in low-back disorders. The rapid and enthusiastic expansion in disc surgery soon exposed its limitations and failures. It was accused of leaving more tragic human wreckage in its wake than any other operation in history."[13]

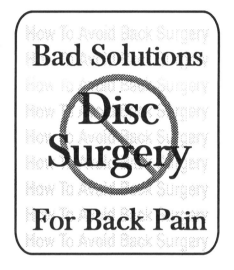

This dramatic increase in back surgeries in the U.S. reminds me of the prophetic statement by the late author Dr. Robert Mendelsohn who said, "The reason why there are 90 percent too many surgeries is because there are 90 percent too many surgeons." The facts clearly indict the medical world and the insurance industry in this conspiracy to exploit the American public. The huge costs of medical care and professional profiteering may be one of the reasons why Congress and the AHCPR took it upon themselves to establish guidelines in this area. Whether or not their guideline will be followed is doubtful as long as the huge fees ($15,000 to $50,000) tempt both surgeons and hospitals alike. Unfortunately in America, money is too often the guiding light in health care nowadays, not research, clinical or ethical considerations.

When the U.S. Public Health Service states that only one in 100 back surgeries for acute low back pain is necessary, something is amiss. It's not just a question of over-utilization for the 99 percent of patients who really didn't need back surgery, it's also a question of the very premise of back surgery itself – that is, that most back pain is due to spinal pathologies such as herniated discs, degenerated discs, bone spurs or some type of spinal arthritis. For decades the medical professionals have equated all back pain to these problems, yet their own research has not supported these contentions. It's one thing to do surgery based on an accurate diagnosis as Dr. Ruth Jackson instructs, but it's another issue to do surgery based on a false premise altogether.

According to Dr. Gordon Waddell in his paper, "Modern Management of Spinal Disorders," presented at the 1995 Chiropractic Centennial Foundation Celebration in Washington, D.C.:

> "Low back pain is a twentieth century health-care disaster. It is now time for a fundamental change in clinical management and re-organization of health-

care to meet the needs of these patients.

"There is a common general criticism that health care for LBP in the U.S. is too specialist-oriented, high-tech, surgical and expensive... At present, too much therapy for LBP consists of symptomatic modalities for pain (Jette et al. 1994), despite the scientific evidence that many of the modalities in common use are ineffective (Spitzer et al. 1987, Bigos et al. 1994). Patients do need symptomatic measures to control pain, but these should be used mainly to facilitate active rehabilitation rather than be seen as an end in themselves.

"There is now considerable evidence that manipulation can be an effective method of providing symptomatic relief for some patients with acute LBP. However manipulation should not be seen in isolation and is only one part of total management. To achieve the desired change in the overall management of simple backache, there should be a fundamental shift in therapy goals and resources to provide active rehabilitation programmes and patient education on prevention and personal responsibility for continued management." [14]

Not the Disc!

In an article titled, "Back Pain: The Best Treatment Is Surprisingly Simple," *Consumer Reports* confirmed that most back pain is not caused by the disc.

"But what, precisely, causes people's lower backs to seize up in pain remains a mystery to this day. Since the 1950s, blame has tended to fall on the discs, the spongy gel-filled cushions between some of the backbones, which can bulge – the familiar herniated or 'slipped' disc. The assumption was that when the bulge pressed on a spinal nerve, it caused back pain.

"Now the assumption is crumbling in the face of new studies showing that when people with no back pain whatever are examined with magnetic resonance imaging scans, about a third of younger adults and virtually all older ones have some bulging discs. In fact, a back full of completely 'normal' discs is the exception, not the rule, even among healthy people. 'Given the high prevalence of these findings and of back pain, the discovery of bulges or protrusions in people with back pain may frequently be coincidental,' conclude the authors of one such study.

"Other possible explanations, also still speculative, are that the lower back muscles somehow go into spasm or that the spinal nerve roots are being compressed by arthritic spurs or bony overgrowth." [15]

Although *Consumer Reports* believes that back pain remains a mystery to the medically-minded whose assumptions were dispelled by the new research, back pain is not a mystery to the thousands of chiropractors who have been treating it for a century with spinal adjustments. The *Consumer Reports* article mentions the fact that the only treatment recommended in the new guideline is spinal manipulation. Since discs, muscles or ligaments cannot be manipulated, it seems that the many joints of the spinal column are the main source of most back pain. It should no longer be a mystery that spinal joint dysfunction is the major cause of back pain. I find it odd that *Consumer Reports* could not come to that same conclusion – obviously their historical prejudice against chiropractic once again just couldn't give credit where credit is due! Although it may be difficult for *Consumer Reports*, the AMA and other medically-minded groups to admit, the new guideline emphatically recommends spinal manipulation as the best initial form of professional treatment for back pain.

The new governmental research studies have exposed once and for all that the "dynasty of the disc," for the most part, has been a huge scientific mistake. Since the 1930s, when two orthopedic surgeons discovered the supposed "slipped disc," back surgeries have typified the "ongoing entrepreneurial misadventure engaged in by orthopedic and neurosurgeons alike" according to Arthur Croft, DC, author of *Whiplash Injuries*, a leading textbook on acceleration/deceleration syndrome. He states, "Despite recent studies that show that the natural history of lumbar disc herniation is to resorb in 67 percent to 78 percent of the cases, and studies that suggest

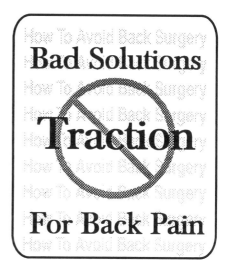

that disc surgery offers no long-term advantage over conservative care, the business of spinal surgery is thriving today, in fact, it is on the increase."[16]

Too often, the medical provider determines the need for back surgery based solely on a positive MRI or myelogram examination which reveals some type of disc abnormality. Whether the disc is swollen, herniated or degenerated is reason enough for most surgeons to warrant a risky surgery. However recently, much evidence has come of light which suggests that too much emphasis is placed on MRI exams, again focusing on disc problems as the main source of pain when in fact, there may be another cause.

In her book, *Disease-Mongers*, author Lynn Payer mentioned a scam that chiropractors have long known – that the so-called "ruptured disc" was a questionable factor in back pain.

> "The rub is that while it's true that most patients suffering back pain can be found to have 'ruptured' discs, once doctors started examining patients who didn't have back pain, they found 'ruptured' discs too. By mid-life 30 to 40 percent of people have them, and in the 60 to 70 age range, 70 to 80 percent of people have a 'ruptured' disc, whether or not they feel, or indeed, ever felt, pain. This, of course, calls into question just what role the ruptured disc plays in causing the backache as well as whether surgery can lessen that pain."[17]

Modern medical researchers from different countries have resoundingly concluded that MRI exams are often misleading. According to Bjorn Rydevik, MD, PhD, of the department of orthopedics, University of Gothenburg, Sweden: "For lumbar disc herniation, it is a well known fact that at least 20-30 percent of all adult individuals have myelographic or MRI evidence of disc herniations without any clinical symptoms."[18] Other researchers found the rate of disc abnormalities to be even higher than 20-30 percent. For instance, a study from the Utah Medical Center in Salt Lake City in 1992 concluded: "With this increased accuracy [of diagnostic testing such as MRI and CT scans] has come recognition of a 50% prevalence of underlying abnormalities in patients between 20 and 60 years old who have no symptoms. When such patients have a back injury, subsequent imaging will show in half of the population studied abnormalities that are not related to an acute injury."[19]

From a 1995 study from George Washington University Medical Center comes more proof of the misplaced emphasis on disc abnormalities as the cause of back pain. "Epidemiologic studies document the overuse of surgical procedures in the United States compared with rates in 11 developed nations...Magnetic resonance imaging findings of intervertebral disc bulging and protrusion occur frequently in asymptomatic individuals."[20] In 1993 another study appeared in the *American Journal of Medical Quality* that stated: "Ninety subjects with complaints of low back pain sustained in a recent motor vehicle accident were studied for their incidence of abnormal findings on lumbar magnetic resonance imaging. The results were compared to other studies reporting a high incidence of abnormal findings on magnetic resonance imaging in asymptomatic subjects. Appropriateness of magnetic resonance imaging in some groups is questioned."[21]

Most recently, in 1995 researchers at the University of Minnesota reviewed MRI studies to investigate whether asymptomatic abnormalities were as common in the thoracic (mid-back) spine as in the lumbar spine. Studies of 90 asymptomatic patients, including 60 patients with no history of back pain and 30 patients who had previous pain in the lower back but not in the thoracic region, were reviewed by researchers who were unaware of the patients' identities and symptoms. Their interpretations of the MRI images revealed that sixty-six of the patients had at least one abnormality; over half had degenerative changes, annular tears, or disc bulges; 37 percent had disc herniations; and 29 percent had deformity of the spinal cord by a protruding disc. There was no obvious correlation between disc abnormalities and age, but men were found to have a higher prevalence of disc bulges and spinal cord deformities than women. The researchers concluded: "This study documents the high prevalence of anatomical irregularities, including herniation of a disc and deformation of the spinal cord, on the magnetic resonance images of the thoracic spine in asymptomatic individuals."[22]

Unnecessary MRI Exams

The gullibility of patients to be overly persuaded by MRI exams typifies Americans' fascination with high-technology equipment. This attraction has allowed many doctors to misuse, misinterpret and mistreat many unsuspecting patients who have blind faith in high-tech exams and in their MDs. This trust mistakenly leads them into many unnecessary procedures that routinely use MRIs. The AHCPR guideline mentions that only one in 200 patients requires this sophisticated testing, yet many more patients each year receive these expensive tests.

Actually, this sentiment was also expressed in the opening remarks by Walter O. Spitzer, MD, of the Quebec Task Force on Whiplash-Related Disorders: "Since World War II, there has been pressure to depend more on sophisticated technology. Such technology often goes through a trendy 'fad phase' and is not always subjected to rigorous scientific evaluation before its use becomes widespread. The price paid by society for such shortcomings is aggravated by procedure-oriented, fee-for-service reimbursement schemes that reward 'doing' much more than 'thinking.'"[23]

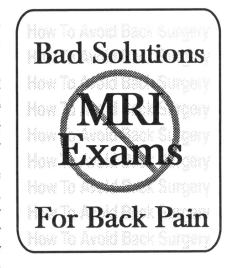

Not only are too many MRI exams routinely performed on back pain patients, but the diagnostic interpretations by radiologists also routinely mistakenly convince patients of the need for surgery when, in fact, they may not require it. In other words, just because an MRI exam is "positive" for some type of disc abnormality, it doesn't mean it is the source of pain nor is surgery required to fix it. As Dr. Scott Boden mentioned about his research, finding disc derangements is like finding gray hair in patients – everyone has them, but it doesn't mean it's the cause of their pain.

The old basic medical premise that back pain is primarily due to disc problems has finally been proven mostly false. For decades the medics have convinced themselves and their patients that all back pain is due to anatomical pathologies – disc derangement, bone spurs or herniation. Despite their high failure rates and new scientific evaluation that disproves this premise, some MDs still refuse to accept the new findings and guideline. And their tunnel-vision has lead too many patients down the road of failed back surgery, chronic pain and pandemic disability. Then again, if your only tool is a hammer, everyone looks like a nail!

In an editorial published in *The New England Journal of Medicine*, a well-known researcher, Dr. Richard A. Deyo made these comments about the overuse of MRI to justify disc surgery:

"The recent increase in the rates of lumbar-spine surgery (laminectomies, discectomies, and fusions) may be related in part to the availability of new imaging techniques. Lumbar surgery is most commonly performed after a herniated intervertebral disc has been diagnosed, often by imaging of the spine. <u>Although surgery relieves pain in carefully selected patients with herniated discs, most patients improve without an operation. Studies suggest that imaging studies only weakly predict either the need for surgery or its outcome</u>...Thus, imaging should be reserved for patients who have signs and symptoms of radiculopathy and who do not have a response to conservative treatment over a period of four to six weeks."[24]

The conservative treatment of which Dr. Deyo speaks is chiropractic spinal manipulation. Unfortunately, most patients are railroaded into unnecessary back surgery on the basis of an MRI exam alone without benefit of first receiving conservative care. If any disc derangement is noted – whether it's swollen, degenerated, bulging, or whatever – most surgeons emphatically agree that it's reason enough to cut. And when patients are in acute pain, the MRI convinces them that the disc is the primary problem and that surgery is the only solution. This is despite the fact that chiropractic adjustments may help in most cases to reduce the herniation. But with pain, fear of disability, and the surgeons' offer of a "quick-fix," most patients consent to these expensive and generally ineffective back surgeries, and are only rarely told of the high failure rates or that chiropractic care can help.

The lack of clinical significance of a "positive" MRI exam is well-known among the medical experts, although it's not being passed on to the public by general practitioners or surgeons who still use a so-called "positive" MRI to convince the gullible patient of the need for surgery. W.P. Butt, MD, of St. James' University Hospital made these comments in the *British Journal of Rheumatology*:

> "There is very little, if any, justifications for MRI scanning in patients with mechanical back pain unless surgery is planned. <u>I know that pretty pictures will be obtained and all sorts of pathological appearances found, but abnormalities are so common in normal asymptomatic individuals of the same age and sex that it is not acceptable to infer that an abnormality is, of itself, significant</u>... Another unfortunate effect of MRI in mechanical back pain results from our gullibility to 'scientific' evidence. We seem to respect an image produced by a computer much more than we respect a shadow. Surgeons who have long since learned not to treat x-rays with surgery will still use surgery to treat a scan... <u>Recently, the president of the Academic Orthopedic Association of the United States stated in his presidential address that 95 percent of spine surgery for back pain was inappropriate.</u> I do not wish to enter into a discussion whether his figures were precise or not, but only to point out that every one of the patients inappropriately operated had pre-operative imaging which was misleading."[25]

The misguided belief that detection of a disc herniation is reason enough to do back surgery was also addressed by the AHCPR report on acute low back pain in adults. Their "Clinical Practice Guideline for Clinicians" clearly mentions this point:

"The presence of a herniated lumbar disc on an imaging study, however, does not necessarily imply nerve root dysfunction. <u>Studies of asymptomatic adults commonly demonstrate intervertebral disc herniations that apparently do not entrap a nerve root or cause symptoms.</u>

"Patients with acute low back pain alone, without findings of serious conditions or significant nerve root compression, rarely benefit from a surgical consultation.

"Many patients with strong clinical findings of nerve root dysfunction due to disc herniation recover activity tolerance within one month; no evidence indicates that delaying surgery for this period worsens outcomes. With or without an operation, more than 80 percent of patients with obvious surgical indications eventually recover. Surgery seems to be a luxury for speeding recovery of patients with obvious surgical indications but benefits fewer than 40 percent of patients with questionable physiologic findings. <u>Moreover, surgery increases the chance of future procedures with higher complications rates.</u> Overall, the incidence of first-time disc surgery complications, including infection and bleeding, is less than 1 percent. The figure increases dramatically with older patients or repeated procedures."[26]

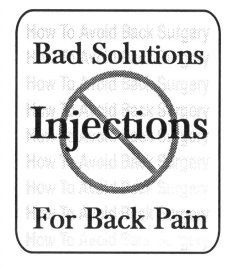

If this research doesn't undermine the basic abnormal disc premise of the medical management of back pain, what more would be convincing enough? Your key to solving this puzzle rests outside the medical arsenal of solutions – it rests with a better, more plausible explanation of altered, dysfunctional spinal mechanics as the source of back pain. As you learn more about how the spine actually works, the chiropractic solution will greatly add to your understanding of this back epidemic. Chiropractors have known for decades that disc problems are secondary to the spinal misalignments and that most back pain is mainly due to joint problems, not disc problems. How else do you explain why some patients with osteoarthritis have no back pain, while others with perfectly healthy spines are full of pain? Because back pain has little to do with disc pathology and everything to do with joint mechanics. This is the fundamental answer to this puzzle of back pain.

Despite the research verifying spinal manipulation's value in helping back pain, the public for the most part naively believes that surgery is the only solution to this problem. Even publication of the article titled, "Ruptured Discs Not Always a Pain," by the Associated Press had little impact on slowing the numbers of unnecessary back surgeries. In fact, if the media wanted to inform the public about dangerous and ineffective procedures, I dare say back surgeries would be an excellent starting point. Instead, the press has been strangely quiet on this important matter. Whistleblowers in the medical world are usually ignored or shouted down, not unlike those brave souls who warn the public about tobacco. Indeed, it seems in the press, that big money speaks the loudest.

The fact that 80 percent of all American adults will suffer from an acute back attack before the age of 50 is a huge problem that has been virtually ignored by the press, and as the research has shown, mostly mismanaged by the medical profession. In fact, back pain is the third largest cause of hospitalization and the number one cause of disability for people under the age of 45. One can only conclude that the main reason for this massive back pain problem rests with the AMA's incessant propaganda against the chiropractic profession. Just as blatant discrimination against the dental profession would have lead to an epidemic of tooth decay and dental problems, the medical profession's illegal discrimination against the chiropractic profession has lead to this massive back pain problem in the U.S. by boycotting and ridiculing the use of spinal manipulation.

Even after the recent investigative reports and media announcements of the new AHCPR guideline, precious little has changed in our country's hospitals and insurance programs to include chiropractic care. The public is still being denied its freedom of choice by the status quo in the health-care delivery system. Instead it is being forced into medical treatment plans with pills, potions and surgery that just don't work. These plans waste millions of dollars, cause untold suffering and disability and result in thousands of cases of failed back surgeries that could have easily been avoided through chiropractic spinal care.

And it's not getting better. My experience is not limited to seeing patients with one failed back surgery; I have seen patients with as many as five and six back surgeries and I have read reports of patients who endured 10 or more surgeries. Even the AHCPR "Clinicians Guide" mentions that the panel found cases where patients underwent as many as 20 failed back surgeries! While the best national researchers emphatically disprove the onslaught of unnecessary back surgery, the costs continue to skyrocket. And we wonder why the back pain epidemic will cost over $100 billion worldwide and nearly $25 in direct medical costs and $75 billion in total costs here in the U.S. annually? Go figure!

The Whole Truth

I always ask every failed back surgery victim why they didn't go to a chiropractor first. Not once have these victims been told there is an alternative to surgery called chiropractic. Although the unethical *voo-doo* diagnosis has been used for decades by too many doctors, given the new research and governmental guideline, these unscrupulous tactics must change, or surgeons will face the risk of malpractice lawsuits. As a patient, it is your legal right to be told of all options for care – even chiropractic care.

Patients are legally entitled to know all possible options of treatment for their conditions. This legal point is intended to help patients get well using the best technology available and to avoid unnecessary and ineffective treatments. All health-care providers must give patients enough information to allow them not just to consent to treatment, but to know about all possible alternatives, enabling what is called "informed consent." A valid, informed consent requires the doctor to advise the patient of many facets of care:

1. The nature of the procedure to be employed.
2. The material risks inherent in the treatment.
3. The probability of those risks occurring.
4. The availability and nature of other treatment options, if any.
5. The material risks inherent in these options and the probability of those risks occurring.
6. The risks and dangers of remaining untreated.

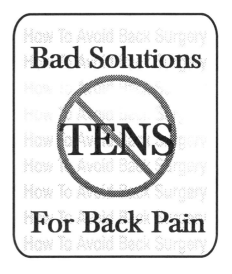

Generally, most MDs fail to live up to their legal responsibility of obtaining informed consent. In fact, they fail to give truthful information to patients asking about chiropractic as an option to surgery. But with the advent of the AHCPR guideline, the federal government has taken on the task of informing the public, proclaiming that spinal manipulation is a viable treatment for acute low back pain in adults. The consumer brochure produced by AHCPR advises the public, *"Your health-care provider may recommend spinal manipulation to help relieve your symptoms."* Furthermore, the guideline states, *"It should only be done by a professional with experience in manipulation."*[27]

Inasmuch as chiropractors perform 94 percent of all manipulation in this country, obviously they are the foremost experts in this field. However, despite this legal issue of informed consent, and despite the endorsement of spinal manipulation by the new federal guideline, many MDs still refuse to afford patients the opportunity to give informed consent. This can be considered illegal as well as an unethical breach of the doctor-patient relationship.

Unfortunately, most MDs continue to ignore the new guideline set forth by the U.S. Public Health Service. A survey by Drs. Daniel Cherkin and Richard Deyo published in *Spine* and titled "Physician Views About Treating Low Back Pain," confirmed the current misinformed medical professionals. Only one in three MDs believes there is any value in spinal manipulation! Furthermore, a majority of U.S. physicians still believe in the effectiveness of treatments *not recommended in the AHCPR guideline,* such as physical therapy (81 percent), bed rest for more than three days (72 percent), and trigger point injections (64 percent). These responses show that MDs are prescribing many of the medical treatments found ineffective by the AHCPR panel, despite their awareness of the guideline. "According to the researchers, less than 3 percent of physicians would order spinal manipulation for any of the hypothetical back pain patients. Ironically, this is the one treatment for which there is substantial evidence for efficacy, especially with acute low back pain." [28] This lack of professional referrals not only drives up medical costs, it drives many patients into unnecessary and ineffective medical care such as surgery.

Let me give you a typical example of a patient whose failed back surgeries stemmed from a questionable disc premise and a lack of informed consent. Recently a prospective patient consulted with me about her constant back pain which persisted despite her having undergone five disc surgeries. After the fifth surgery, she asked her neurosurgeon why she still hurt as "bad as I did before the first surgery." He was perplexed because, as he told her, "I got all the disc." Because he is a highly skilled surgeon, I'm sure he did get all the disc material. But if the disc was the source of pain, why did she still hurt? Good question – one that must baffle many patients with failed back surgery syndrome. When I told her, "Perhaps it's not the disc causing your back pain," it was like hitting her with a brick! She was stunned, to say the least!

I asked the patient if she was aware that there are 137 joints in the human spine, and that misalignments of these joints are the cause of most all back pain. "He never mentioned that possibility," she replied. Can you imagine how she felt when shortly thereafter the Associated Press reprinted an account of Dr. Maureen Jensen's article from *The New England Journal of Medicine,* suggesting that disc abnormalities are not the cause of back pain? Can you imagine how the hundreds of thousands of patients with failed back surgeries must feel when they learn that their surgeries were based on a false premise, experimental at best and unnecessary and ineffective at worse?

Obviously, spinal pathology is not the key to solving the epidemic of back problems. Although chiropractors have been stating this very fact for decades and have been virtually ignored, this new supportive research will nonetheless be slow to change anything in the medical world. In fact, according to the Office of Technology Assessment (OTA), the hope that research into medical effectiveness by the federal government will change the present exploitative system is overly optimistic. A report by OTA stated that, "passive dissemination of guidelines to clinicians, however, often has no effect" in changing clinical practice. The status quo in health care is less interested in clinical effectiveness than it is interested in maintaining its complete control over health-care dollars. In addition, if a patient were aware of Drs. Boden and Jensen's research, his or her personal physician probably would deny the study's validity, just as they have routinely denied the effectiveness of chiropractic care. How can any patient trust an MD who would lie about this important and pervasive problem? And the AMA wonders why their image is at its lowest ebb in years, and we wonder why we have an epidemic of failed back surgery?

The facts are clear: The chiropractic approach has proven vastly superior to the medical model, yet there are some MDs who refuse to accept the truth because they might not profit. Inasmuch as 70 percent of the average neurosurgeon's income comes from back surgeries, and since back attacks are the third most common reason for hospital admissions, the medical profession's inertia allows it to stay the present expensive course, despite the recent new findings. But this course will have to change soon. It's one thing for chiropractors, researchers or a few honest surgeons to say 99 percent of back surgeries are unnecessary, but when the U.S. Public Health Service agrees, the medical boat will have to change course. When the new AHCPR guideline is implemented and legally enforced after a few malpractice cases, it should turn the entire back pain industry upside-down. Patients no longer will be routinely fed the standard medical procedure of bed rest, pain drugs, hot packs, MRI exams and back surgery – all of which are now considered mostly ineffective and expensive methods. Instead, the new guideline directs patients first to receive hot/ice packs (I recommend ice, not hot packs), acetaminophen or NSAIDs and spinal manipulation.

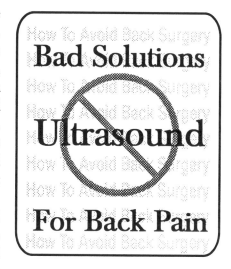

Can you imagine the impact this will have when chiropractors are seeing a majority of patients with back pain instead of seeing just the few people who are aware of chiropractic or only seeing the "last resorts" from the medical world? The cost reductions will be enormous and the patient satisfaction rate will also be just as huge. I've long believed that patients don't know how good they can feel until they've had their spines adjusted. Furthermore, the insurance companies don't realize how much money they can save by using chiropractic care first in the management of back pain. While the winners will certainly be the patients and their insurance payers, the only losers will be the surgeons and hospitals who have exploited the public for too long with ineffective and expensive back surgeries.

The Real Cause of Most Back Pain

Considering that the medical model of pulled muscles and slipped discs simply isn't true for the vast majority of back injuries, you may wonder why has the medical model been so ineffective for back pain? What the medical world has forgotten to ask is: Why do the discs herniate? While the 23 intervertebral discs are involved, they remain a secondary problem. No disc will herniate, swell, rupture or degenerate on its own volition – discs only become symptomatic and pathological when the structure of the spinal column forces them to deviate from their normal, painless function. The simple fact that the spinal column – the 24 vertebrae sitting on top of 3 pelvic bones – is inter-connected by 137 joints is the main consideration routinely omitted in their explanations to patients.

Obviously, the facts show that the disc model of back pain hasn't proven clinically or cost-effective. But why? If a disc herniation is the main problem, removing it sounds reasonable, doesn't it? And when the MRI shows the disc bulge, isn't that proof enough to warrant surgery? Apparently not, and for good reason. The disc problem has proven to be a secondary problem in the back pain scenario. Obviously a disc doesn't protrude because it wants to on its own; it does so only when it's forced to move, mainly due to spinal misalignments – or in chiropractic parlance – vertebral subluxations.

When the spine is misaligned, the interconnecting disc between the vertebrae is forced to wedge or bulge to the wide side of the misalignment. This bulge is the herniation that is seen on the MRI. It is simply a secondary response to the misalignment of the vertebrae. Simply removing the offending disc bulge may seem logical and may give momentary relief in some cases, but if the spinal vertebrae joints remain misaligned, no significant correction has occurred. Again, it's simply treating the symptom of the problem and not correcting the underlying cause. Perhaps this explains why the AHCPR experts concluded that only one in 100 back surgeries is helpful.

Chiropractors know that misaligned spinal joints are considered to be the main source of most back pain, not swollen discs or pulled muscles, and that's why spinal manipulation has always worked so well. Considering that there are 137 joints in the human spinal column, you can see how accidents, falls or sitting all day long can compress, twist or misalign these joints. Whenever normal joint motion is lost, the resultant damage is pain, stiffness, disc swelling and nerve pressure, and if this condition is not corrected by spinal adjustments, spinal arthritis eventually results from an acute condition becoming chronic. Simply removing a protruding disc without realigning the spinal joints will not remove the main source of pain. It is easy to understand why the vast majority of back surgeries fail, because they are addressing a secondary problem and not the primary issue of spinal joint misalignments.

Most doctors forget that the disc is not the only point of contact between vertebrae. There are three points – the disc and the two posterior facet joints. The posterior facets are richly innervated with pain-sensitive nerve fibers, much more so than the disc, which has nerve supply only to the outer third of the annulus. Even though joint dysfunction cannot be seen on an x-ray or an MRI, it nonetheless is the primary source of pain in most back attacks. This explains why disc surgery often fails – if the main source of pain is the facet joints, surgery to remove the herniated or degenerated disc will be of little help. Actually, altering the disc height through removal will only add to the problem by creating more joint dysfunction.

Ironically, there have been no randomized controlled studies for many of the most common spinal surgeries, such as neck fusions or laminectomy, an operation performed over 20,000 times each year. According to Dr. Nikolai Bogduk in his paper, "The Anatomical Basis for Spinal Pain Syndromes," back pain is primarily due to joint dysfunction and not disc abnormalities or pulled muscles:

44

"There are no scientific data, however, that sustain the belief that muscles may be a source of chronic pain... cervical zygapophysial joint pain accounts for more than 50 percent of all instances of chronic neck pain following whiplash based on controlled studies using comparative local anesthetic blocks... Cervical discography may be falsely positive in over 40 percent of cases...In another study, 50 percent of patients with cervical myelopathy reported positive responses to discopathy, yet none had ever suffered neck pain.

"...Of all the various therapies for neck pain, only early manual therapy for whiplash has been vindicated in the literature."[29]

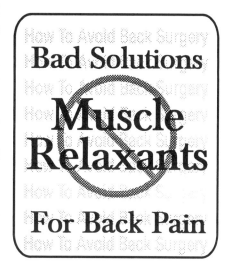

Growing numbers of experienced medical manipulators now adopt a similar approach to back pain as chiropractors have long utilized. According to both John F. Bourdillon, MD, and E.A. Day, MD:

"There is no doubt that the symptoms of some patients with actual disc protrusions do improve with manipulative treatment... It appears that the softening and subsequent protrusion of disc material is a complication of spinal joint dysfunction... only in some patients does it interfere with recovery enough to justify removal.

"The sacroiliac joint appears to be the single greatest cause of back pain. the range of motion is small and difficult to describe but, when normal joint play is lost, agonizing pain can be precipitated... (the sacroiliac) joints are complex and not fully understood, but it is clear to the authors that they can have a profound effect on body mechanics... anyone who still holds the view that these joints are immobile can never hope to achieve control of common back pain." [30]

The research about the effectiveness of manipulation and the ineffectiveness of back surgery has been well known by many health professionals for years. No longer are these revelations only coming from remote researchers and "alternative" practitioners, they now are the conclusions of the British, Canadian and U.S. governmental researchers.

Consider these comments again from Dr. John Bourdillon, trained in orthopedic surgery and manipulation at St. Thomas' Hospital, London, author of the text *Spinal Manipulation* and past president of the North American Academy of Manipulative Medicine:

"My interest in the other schools of manipulative therapy was stimulated by a number of patients whose backs I had treated without success, who were kind enough to let me know that subsequent visits to non-medically qualified manipulators had given satisfactory results... One of the patients was a woman whose low lumbar spine I had explored on two occasions and from whom I had removed disc protrusions at both the lumbo-sacral joint and the L4/L5 joint. In spite of this she was still crippled by severe symptoms. Dr. Turner, a chiropractor, succeeded in relieving her and I continued to treat her for many years afterwards when she had recurrences.

"The main trouble in her case was a sciatic radiation of pain caused by a sacroiliac strain and I well remember my bland feeling of disbelief when Dr. Turner suggested this possibility. 'How', I said to myself, 'can the sacroiliac joint possibly cause a sciatica when there is no conceivable means by which any of the nerves of the sacral plexus can be pressed on by such a joint strain?' Dr. Turner's results and my subsequent experience have, for me, completely proved that a sacroiliac strain can be the cause of a sciatica, but the precise means by which this pain reference is produced remains a matter of theory for which adequate experimental proof is still lacking." [31]

In another similar experience, Hubert Rosomoff, MD, neurosurgeon and chairman of the Department of Neurological Surgery at the University of Miami, was one of several surgeons who illustrated the dramatic change in medical management of low back pain. Earlier in his career, he operated on several thousand patients with back and leg pain on the model of relieving nerve root compression from supposed disc herniation. With growing experience he decided that disc herniation, even when clearly visible through MRI imaging, was seldom the cause of pain. "Pain is from a passing impulse, not a continuing compression. We know a lot about peripheral pain but very little about the cause of deep tissue pain – pain in the muscles and ligaments."

Concluding that "back pain should be viewed as a non-surgical problem, subject to a few exceptions," Dr. Rosomoff imposed a moratorium on surgery at his hospital. His subsequent extensive non-surgical experience has convinced him that "a simple medical back examination is no good...the underlying problem is usually missed...all chronic low back pain is an iatrogenic disability because of the unskilled medical diagnosis and management...the herniated disc doesn't produce pain, per se, and the most common cause of pain is associated with muscle damage." Asked what use he made of traditional muscle relaxants, Dr. Rosomoff replied: "Generally none – there is no evidence that muscle relaxants will help mechanical contraction of muscle."[32]

Unfortunately for most medical patients, the first approach to any back pain by most MDs is the simple remedy of pain pills and muscle relaxants despite their obvious failings. The Manga Report mentions that almost half of all MDs (47%) still believe the major reason for low back pain was "muscle strain." These researchers also found patients' dissatisfaction with the information they received from their MDs about their back pain:

"Patients of family physicians were significantly less satisfied than patients of chiropractors with the information they received about their back problem, including the cause of the back pain, recovery time, content of care and instructions on exercise, posture and lifting...Physicians' patients were also significantly much less confident in the correctness of the diagnosis, or in the effectiveness of treatment; and in the comfort with which the provider was in dealing with the patients' complaint of back pain."[33]

The overuse of muscle relaxants – a common medical solution to back pain – is not without governmental criticism as well. In the AHCPR guideline on acute low back pain, the *Quick Reference Guide for Clinicians* clearly states the ineffectiveness of such drugs: "The therapeutic objective of muscle relaxants is to reduce low back pain by relieving muscle spasm. However, the concept of skeletal muscle spasm is not universally accepted as a cause of symptoms, and the most commonly used muscle relaxants have no peripheral effect on muscle spasm."[34]

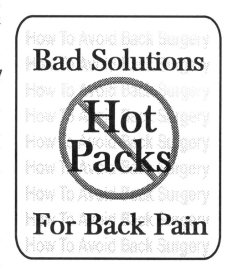

An article in the *Scandinavian Journal of Rehabilitation Medicine* by C. Pedersen titled "Management of Spasticity on Neurophysiological Basis," confirmed that a simple ice pack can completely alleviate a muscle spasm and its pain within 10 to 20 minutes.[35] And an ice pack is much less expensive and less prone to harmful side effects than drugs. As every chiropractor knows, not only will ice packs reduce muscle spasm temporarily, but removing nerve pressure will reduce the spasm by correcting the underlying cause. Muscle fibers contract involuntarily when spinal misalignments irritate the nerve roots causing the muscle to spasm. Although ice therapy is more effective than drug therapy, a chiropractic adjustment is the best therapy of all to help this problem.

Questionable Recommendations

The low back pain guideline from the AHCPR panel did make a few conclusions that I felt were questionable, but which are typical of a medical symptomatic orientation toward any pain problem. First of all, the researchers state that 90 percent of acute low back pain will resolve itself within a month and recommend that patients use ice/hot packs and acetaminophen or NSAIDs, and if that failed, to visit a *"health professional"* for spinal manipulation. Although many bouts of back pain may diminish within a month, just "waiting it out" is no answer to the problem. That's like waiting out a toothache by masking it with pain pills or hoping your chest pains will just go away on their own.

Again, the medical researchers seemed more concerned about controlling pain than correcting the underlying cause of the problem. In fact, masking any symptom with ice packs and acetaminophen or NSAIDs will only serve to make an acute problem a chronic one. Even a disc surgery merely treats the symptom. Don't think for a moment that these symptomatic medical approaches have changed anything permanently. Although it is common with a medical approach, living through the pain or masking symptoms is no way to manage back pain. Perhaps this approach explains why 70 percent of back pain patients relapse within six months, according to spinal expert Dr. Gordon Waddell.[36]

The AHCPR guideline also recommends hot packs or ice therapy to control back pain. Although the use of hot packs is commonplace, it generally causes more problems by increasing the internal swelling. As you know, heat by nature expands tissues, so putting a hot pack on a back injury will increase the internal pressure, causing it to swell more, and creating more pain in the long run. On the other hand, ice by nature shrinks tissues and numbs the nerves. I recommend using ice exclusively for 30 minutes every hour, if necessary. If there is absolutely no swelling, such as in an old injury, heat may be appropriate, but for any new problem stay with ice packs.

The guideline also recommends using over-the-counter (OTC) drugs instead of prescriptions drugs which have stronger side-effects. While that is good advice, using OTC drugs for prolonged periods does not make good sense when other research has revealed their dangers. Researchers at the University of Pittsburgh found that people may suffer liver damage if they are too sick to eat and take a moderate overdose of acetaminophen (Tylenol) – 8 to 20 tablets – within a 24-hour period. In another study at John Hopkins University, it was determined that arthritis sufferers who take acetaminophen every day for a year raise their risk of kidney failure by about 40 percent. Even simple aspirin has been proven to cause intestinal bleeding and macular degeneration. In fact, the U.S. Food and Drug Administration estimates that 10,000 to 20,000 people die each year from stomach problems caused by NSAID use.[37]

Clearly, even relatively "safe" drugs have their serious side-effects. Again, the answer to pain control is not masking it with pain pills of any type or strength. The real answer is to correct the underlying cause of the problem, which pills can never do. The real answer is to stabilize your spinal problem with chiropractic care and spinal exercises.

Official Medical Misinformation About Back Pain

Another glaring illustration of the AMA's refusal to acknowledge research and treatments from which they will not profit, is their May 1995 publication titled, "AMA Pocket Guide to Back Pain," published by Random House.[38] In their attempt to once again confuse the public about the best methods for back pain treatment, the AMA propagandists decided to ignore the AHCPR guideline and to perpetuate their old, ineffective methods which are profitable to many surgeons.

The cover of the pocket guide claims it contains: *"The latest information on all treatment options, including medications, physical therapy and surgery."* Despite the fact that chiropractic spinal manipulation is now the preferred initial form of professional treatment endorsed by the U.S., U.K. and Canadian studies, no mention is ever made of this form of care. The word "chiropractic" is not even mentioned in the entire pocket guide! Yet the AMA claims it includes *"information on all treatment options."* Furthermore, their guide includes many recommendations that contradict the findings of the AHCPR panel. For example:

1. There is no mention whatsoever of spinal manipulation, which is perhaps the mainstay of the AHCPR guideline.

2. *"Bedrest may be necessary for a few days or a few weeks"* – totally contradicts the guideline's recommendations for a return to activity as soon as possible.

3. *"Corticosteroid drugs, such as cortisone, are especially effective in decreasing inflammation."* The AMA guide also supports the use of both injections and oral corticosteroids – methods which the AHCPR panel found expensive and ineffective.

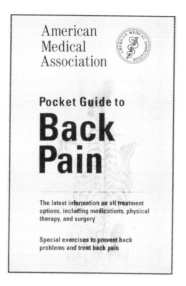

4. Both muscle relaxants and anti-depressants are encouraged by the AMA. *"If your back pain is caused by muscle spasms... your physicians may prescribe muscle relaxants... Other medications frequently used to relieve back pain are anti-depressants which not only improve sleep and mood but are very good at providing pain relief."* Again, the theory of muscle spasm as a source of back pain was disproved by the AHCPR panel, and drugs were rejected as a solution.

5. *"A high percentage of discectomies and fusions are successful in relieving pain."* The AMA guidebook fails to give real statistics to support its unfounded claim while the AHCPR consumer version clearly states that only one in 100 back surgeries is helpful!

6. The AMA also understates the dangers of paralysis from surgery by stating, *"This is a small but real risk, especially with surgery in the cervical (neck) region."* What they fail to state is that the rate is 15,000 cases of paralysis per million!

Ironically, this so-called expert guidebook contains glaring errors that any high school student would notice, such as its description of the spine itself: *"The spine is a structural wonder. A skeletal column formed by 33 bones called vertebrae, the spine supports the body's weight."* The fact is there are only <u>24</u> vertebrae in the human spine! Perhaps the AMA's experts have discovered a few more vertebrae in the human spine? This guidebook also mentions that only *"one joint attaches the spine to the skull,"* another glaring mistake. In fact, the Atlas vertebrae has <u>two</u> joints which articulate with the skull, not one.

Its description of the spine also mentions that: *"More than 100 separate joints connect the bones of the spine to each other and to other bones. Seventy-six facet joints attach the vertebrae to each other, 24 joints connect the thoracic vertebrae to the ribs, two joints connect the sacrum to the hips, and one joint attaches the spine to the skull. "*

It came as a surprise to me that the AMA's description would even mention the fact that the spine is connected together by a multitude of joints, implying to readers the great possibility of joint dysfunction as a source of back pain. In its discussion of the main causes of low back pain, of course, the guide focuses primarily upon the outdated concepts of "pulled muscles" and "slipped discs." However, it does include the possibility of joint problems as a cause: *"Facet joint displacement occurs when twisting movements of the spine cause two vertebrae to slip and lock out of place at a facet joint. Again, the displaced vertebrae may press on a nerve root. Both prolapsed disc and facet joint displacement often cause spasms in the muscles overlying the affected joint. This increases the pain. "*

Again, while these experts admit that joint problems can be the cause of back pain, no mention is made of correcting this type of problem through spinal manipulation. Initially, I thought the AMA at least would admit that joint problems are a big cause of pain, just to be in agreement with other researchers. I presumed they would recommend seeking the help of a physical therapist, osteopath or a medical doctor who attempts spinal manipulation. But this guidebook doesn't even suggest this alternative – it implies that spinal manipulation just doesn't exist as an alternative treatment whatsoever!

It appears quite odd that six months after the conclusion of the most extensive study on back pain ever conducted in our country, the AMA would print a guidebook that totally refutes the AHCPR panel's advice. Is it just coincidental that the AMA published such drivel, or is it another example of medical misinformation to confuse the public? It seems obvious that the AMA is willing to ignore research that conflicts with its own vested interests and to misrepresent the truth despite the harm it will cause patients who follow its ineffective advice. Ironically, in its guidebook, the AMA has the audacity to refer to itself as *"The Nation's Most Trusted Health Care Authority. "* Unfortunately, some readers will believe this medical misinformation and suffer the consequences of failed back surgery. And we wonder why we have an epidemic of back pain and why Dr. Gordon Waddell considers low back pain a 20th century health-care disaster?

Comparing Apples to Oranges

Another glaring example of medical misinformation promoted by the news media appeared in an October 5, 1995 article in *The New England Journal of Medicine,* written by Tim Carey, MD, MPH, et al., from the North Carolina Back Pain Project.[39] The article, titled, "The Outcomes and Costs of Care for Acute Low Back Pain Among Patients Seen by Primary Care Practitioners, Chiropractors and Orthopedic Surgeons," illustrates the depths to which medical misinformants will stoop to confuse the public about the best and cheapest type of care.

The authors did conclude that "Patients who saw chiropractors reported a significantly higher degree of satisfaction than those who saw practitioners in the other four strata." These researchers also concluded that the time to recovery was essentially the same and that chiropractic care was the most costly because of the extended treatment plan of spinal manipulation, which averaged 10 to 15 visits, whereas the medical patients made only two to three visits. Of course, the treatment offered by the MD group was comprised solely of pain medication, muscle relaxants and narcotic agents, none of which are suggested by the AHCPR guideline on acute low back pain in adults.

Ironically, although orthopedic surgeons were involved in this comparison, not one back surgery was performed or factored into this study! As Dr. Carey mentioned in his study, "Because of the low number of hospitalizations, we focused on outpatient charges." Is it little wonder that without considering the huge costs of surgery and hospitalization the medical groups costs were less than the chiropractic group? Comparing drug therapy with chiropractic spinal rehabilitation is the equivalent of comparing apples and oranges! Certainly, simply taking pills is cheaper than any other type of care, but the real crux of this issue – correcting the underlying cause – was not factored into this study. And to exclude the expenses of back surgery in this study is outright, fraudulent misrepresentation of a true comparison. Considering MetLife's statistics on average charges – $7,120 for non-surgical and $13,990

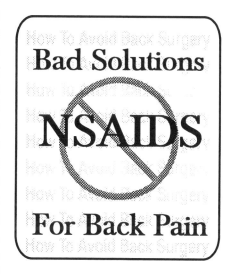

for surgical back cases – and yet, these researchers had the gall to suggest that chiropractic care is more expensive when they omitted the most flagrant expense in this $100 billion health-care disaster – back surgery!

This is just another example of the AMA using the media to misrepresent the truth about back pain care to the public. Hopefully, the public can see this as a case of comparing apples to oranges and as a study that was flawed from the beginning to discount the findings from other more notable research studies (Koes,[40] Jarvis,[41] Wolk,[42] Schifrin,[43] Dean[44]) which emphatically prove that chiropractic care is cheaper than the medical management of back pain. Unfortunately, few people are aware of the research that proves chiropractic is less expensive, and the medically-biased insurance companies will use Dr. Carey's flawed study to exclude chiropractic from their coverage, which was exactly the hidden agenda behind this controversial study.

As a practitioner, I was stunned to learn that these researchers actually believe that masking pain and symptoms is equivalent to correcting the underlying cause of joint dysfunction. That's like equating aspirin with heart surgery as a treatment for chest pain. Apparently, the medical goal of these researchers was simply to mask the pain and not to correct the real cause of the problem – typical of medical mismanagement that often turns acute cases into chronic ones. In this study, the researchers noted that at the end of six months, 31 percent of the patients had not recovered completely; yet there is no data that indicates which type of treatment was used on these failures. Perhaps this omission was to "save face" for the medical treatment of pills that failed to correct the real cause of the subjects' back pain. Just remember: Taking pain pills for back pain is equivalent to taking aspirin for a toothache – while it may temporarily mask the pain, it does nothing to correct the underlying cause. Unfortunately, this flawed study suggests this very approach to the management of back pain.

Let these two examples of medical misinformation – the "AMA Pocket Guide to Back Pain" and this flawed study from the North Carolina Back Pain Project – be a warning to you that you just cannot trust the medical authorities to give you the whole truth about this epidemic of back pain. Unless you're aware of the facts, these distortions of legitimate research will sway you to depend on useless drugs and risky back surgeries – which is exactly the goal of the AMA. Consumer beware!

Victims of "The System"

But what happens to the person who follows the medical doctor's advice and becomes one of the thousands of failed back surgery victims each year? Considering that in 1992 just over 300,000 back surgeries were performed in the U.S., and that according to many honest neurosurgeons and medical researchers as many as 90 percent of these surgeries were unnecessary and ineffective, many patients are in dire straits, to say the least. The tragedy of these failed surgeries is not just wasted money, but often wasted lives and permanent disability.

Let me give you a few examples of victims of "the system." A few years ago, a middle-aged lady presented herself at my office complaining of a mild sore neck from a low-speed car accident. Actually, her car was bumped while it was stopped at a red light by a truck whose driver simply let his foot off the brake too early. The collision was so minor it didn't even dent either bumper, and the lady came to my office with a mild case of neck pain and stiffness. After a short spinal adjustment program, I dismissed her case with a clean bill of health. Around 18 months later, the attorney for the truck driver's insurance company came by my office to discuss her case. Apparently, since I last saw her, this lady had undergone three back surgeries, two on her neck and one on her low back. I was astounded to learn this, inasmuch as she was OK when she left my care and she never once had complained about her low back. Also, her attorney was suing for over a quarter of a million dollars!

When I telephoned her attorney I squarely asked him how this could have happened. He told me he had sent his client to a neurosurgeon who discovered she had degenerative disc disease in her neck and low back. Regardless of the fact that the patient had no back pain, the surgeon used this chronic disc disease as reason enough to cut. After three surgeries, the lady was in worse pain than ever before, and now she was partially disabled from the surgeries. After learning of this ill-begotten affair between the attorney and surgeon, I was willing to testify that all three surgeries were unnecessary. Instead of the quarter of a million dollars she expected, she settled out of court for a mere $90,000. Her attorney got his $30,000 and her surgeon got his $45,000. All this lady got out of the deal was a permanent back disability and some cash. In retrospect, I wonder if she now thinks her three unnecessary back surgeries were worth the few thousand dollars she won, along with a permanently surgically-impaired spine?

Another interesting example of how "the system" fails to provide patients with the basis for informed consent involved a head nurse at a local hospital. She complained of intense back pain and sciatica down one leg. After two disc surgeries she got some relief from her leg pain, but her back pain was still intense and she could sleep only 45 minutes a night before awakening from the pain. After two years of this unrelenting pain, she finally came to my office. I diagnosed a sacroiliac misalignment as the main cause of her low back pain, and after only a few adjustments her pain was diminished and she was able to sleep through the night. She was overjoyed, to say the least.

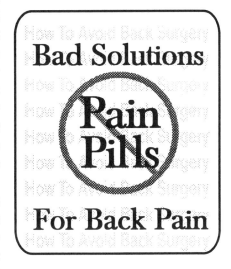

But her employers weren't. I have an "infomercial" about chiropractic which runs on a local cable television station, and my patient volunteered to appear to tell her story. Apparently, the head of the hospital where she worked saw the cable program and confronted her about her testimonial appearance. She told him of her poor response to surgery, her inability to sleep at night and her quick recovery with chiropractic care. Then she asked him why chiropractic care wasn't available in the hospital and why patients aren't informed of this viable alternative to surgery. Of course, her inquiries fell on deaf ears and despite her good recovery, the administrator frowned at her and informed her that if she continued to appear on television praising chiropractic, her job might be in jeopardy. As she told me this story, it reminded me that in the medical world there are *right* and *wrong* ways to get well!

Not only are the discriminatory physicians and hospital administrators to blame for this epidemic, but so is the insurance industry which has chosen to ignore the scientific research and to boycott or limit chiropractic coverage. Often patients are railroaded into back surgeries because their health insurance fails to cover chiropractic care.

As an example of this fact, another patient presented himself at my office complaining of a severe low back attack. His medic had ordered an MRI which showed a disc herniation at L5, where 90 percent of all low back pain occurs. Of course, immediate back surgery was recommended, but the patient didn't want to go that route, so he came to see me. My analysis showed that his disc herniation was due to a spinal misalignment in the same area. After a few weeks of adjustments, this satisfied patient was completely free of pain, never lost any time at work and lives without any permanent problems or disability.

When my office submitted the bill to his insurance carrier, we received a telephone call from the claims adjustor, who questioned my treatment plan, attempted to discredit our care and cut the cost. My conversation with this adjustor was a typical one, because most adjustors are taught to cut chiropractic claims routinely. So I asked the adjustor if he routinely cut the neurosurgeon's bill. "Of course not," he replied. I told him I was confused. If I was able to return this man to work, fully functional and without any added costs or permanent impairment, what was the problem? My bill was less than one tenth the cost of a standard back surgery. Not only that, since I cured the patient of a severe problem, one that supposedly warranted surgery, why wasn't I due the same reward as the neurosurgeon? "Because you're not a surgeon," he replied. I responded to him by saying that my means shouldn't matter if I achieved the same positive end result. "If I can use better technology without the need of invasive surgery or dangerous drugs, why aren't I given the same reward?" The point is simply this: My means to the end shouldn't be an issue, as long as I achieved the same good result.

I also asked the claims adjustor if he was aware that 90 percent of all back surgeries are ineffective. He wouldn't admit to that high percentage, but he did confess that many patients had recurring back surgeries and never seemed to get well. When I read that the insurance industry is looking for ways to decrease costs, and yet it discriminates against the chiropractic profession, which is now considered cheaper, quicker, safer and better by the researchers, I have to think they are less than genuine in their pleas. Again, it seems the insurance industry would rather pay surgeons for clinically ineffective back surgeries than pay chiropractors a fraction of that cost for better clinical results. Again, it's simply the tyranny of "the system."

Let me illustrate the outright absurdity that goes on behind the public's back. A patient of mine who is an operating room nurse in a local hospital came to me with neck and arm pain. She had tried the pain pills and muscle relaxants, but they failed to help her. She didn't want neck surgery because she worked with the local neurosurgeons who performed them. Initially she was quite skeptical of chiropractic, but within a few weeks of receiving spinal adjustments she was feeling great. It was then that she confessed to me a startling revelation: "Half the time when a patient is having a back surgery, the doctors open up the patient, see that the disc is not herniated, turn to each other and have a good laugh and then they do the surgery anyway." I was shocked at her admission and asked, "If the disc isn't ruptured, why don't they sew the patient back up and stop?" She looked at me like I was the fool and said, "Would you pass up $15,000 when you already have the patient convinced and he'll never know the difference?" I simply shook my head and responded, "Sorry, I just let my ethics get in the way."

Unfortunately, this scenario is replayed every day in our country. The typical medical routine consists of using an MRI to validate a disc herniation and to warrant surgery, although new research completely refutes this idea. No one questions the surgeon's opinion. Meanwhile, the insurance industry, the hospitals and the press all stand by without comment. And we wonder why we have an epidemic of failed back surgery when patients are routinely railroaded into unnecessary surgery by "the system."

Putting the Screws to Patients

Another example of gross medical mismanagement of a back injury occurred when a patient appeared in my clinic complaining of increasing back pain, despite having undergone six back surgeries. After the first five attempts at spinal fusion failed, the same surgeon decided to put spinal pedicle screws into the patient's vertebrae. These screws have never been approved by the FDA for such usage. When this radical surgery also failed, the patient finally came to me as a last resort. Not only did these six surgeries cost plenty, the patient also incurred expenses with drug rehab from the medications, physical rehab and other customary hospitalization costs associated with these surgeries. All totaled, he told me his case had cost the state Workers' Compensation program $1.3 million, and he still was hurting just as badly as before his first surgery.

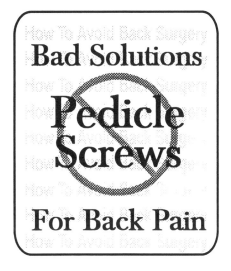

After conducting a chiropractic spinal analysis, I could easily detect his problem. Rather than being a messy situation, the problem turned out to be a rather routine spinal situation – one leg was one-half inch shorter than the other, causing a sacral tilt and a minor lumbar curvature. As I told the patient, a small, inexpensive heel lift and an average spinal adjustment program could possibly have avoided six failed back surgeries, permanent disability and $1.3 million in expenses. As I have found through working with hundreds of failed back surgery cases, this example is not the exception, but rather the rule. The medics simply have ignored the obvious and jumped into these expensive surgeries to no avail.

The use of pedicle screws has come under increasing criticism by chiropractors and consumer groups as well. More than 1,000 Americans a week have steel screws implanted in their spines to fight back pain, although the devices are not government-approved and studies show they may cause more harm than good, according to Sidney Wolfe, MD, of the consumer advocate group, Public Citizen, headed by Ralph Nader. As many as 50-70,000 people receive this treatment every year for such common ailments as chronic low back pain which generally can be managed with manipulation and exercise. In December 1994, Public Citizen released its own investigation of the screws, concluding that they endanger thousands, that the FDA has been negligent in fighting their illegal promotion and that they are pushed by surgeons who receive profitable stock shares in return. "We found evidence of manufacturers' aggressive, illegal marketing of a dangerous device, often with the complicity of co-opted surgeons," said Public Citizen attorney Joanne Mott.[45]

Her review of medical studies found that spinal screws cause complications in one-third of all patients and break off inside the spine in 10 percent of cases. Also, screw recipients are twice as likely to need additional spinal operations than are patients who undergo traditional surgery to fuse their spinal bones without screws, according to Mott's report. Yet patients aren't told that the devices are experimental. Her survey of 101 screw recipients found only one who recalled being told that the device was not FDA-approved. As well, the FDA never took any action against the seven manufacturers it warned to stop advertising spinal screws. As proof, Mott sent the FDA copies of full-page ads for the screws, all published in respected health journals and made by seven different manufacturers. So far the FDA has chosen to ignore this problem, and the use of pedicle screws in back surgery continues unabated, despite their failings and dangers.

The use of spinal screws is yet another example of the medical mismanagement of our nation's back problems. While spinal fusions, discectomies and spinal pedicle screws may be necessary and effective in rare instances (about one in 100 cases), the vast majority of these patients can be helped with chiropractic care instead. Just as most surgical patients are not informed about the danger of the screws, I dare say they also are not informed about chiropractic care as an alternative either. Undoubtedly, they probably are given the *voo-doo* diagnosis about chiropractic instead – *"If you don't have my surgery you'll get worse, and if you go to a chiropractor, he'll paralyze you."* Perhaps patients who fell for this medical *voo-doo* now can see that they have been screwed, literally and figuratively, by their surgeons.

It is interesting to note that the AHCPR guideline for acute low back pain was delayed for months in a court battle by a group of orthopedic surgeons and the manufacturers of these spinal screws. Apparently they didn't like the conclusions of the 23-member expert panel that failed to recommend their experimental methods. Despite the fact that the expert panel criticized the screws, a federal court rejected the defendants' plea, a consumer group called for the end of their usage and more than 600 patients have joined a class action lawsuit, the FDA and the insurance industry have done little to stop this surgical predation upon patients. Despite warnings by the FDA, some surgeons have chosen to experiment upon patients with these radical surgeries that, for the most part, could have been prevented with chiropractic care. As Dr. Wolfe demanded, "This has got to stop. It is a major and dangerous racket being perpetuated on patients in this country." Chiropractors know this only too well, because we see these medical failures every day in our offices.

The news release by Dr. Wolfe and Public Citizen mentioned that pedicle screw surgery is tremendously profitable for everyone involved: manufacturers, orthopedic and neurosurgeons, neurologists, hospitals and radiologists. "There seems to be a conspiracy of silence about the risks among members of industry and much of the medical and hospital communities because of the profitability and fear of litigation. The Orthopedic Surgery community has threatened to blackball any surgeon who speaks against the use of pedicle screws." [46]

Again, we wonder why we have an epidemic of back pain when ethical MDs are intimidated to tell the public the truth. Apparently some honest MDs are victims of "the system" as well.

When Is Back Surgery Necessary?

According to the AHCPR guideline, there are occasions when back surgery is necessary; however they are far less frequent than the average surgeon would agree. Actually, the guideline states that only one in 200 cases of acute low back pain needs extensive testing like MRI exams and that only one in 100 back surgeries is helpful:

> "Patients with acute low back pain alone, without findings of serious conditions or significant nerve root compression, rarely benefit from a surgical consultation. Many patients with strong clinical findings of nerve root dysfunction due to disc herniation recover activity tolerance within one month; no evidence indicates that delaying surgery for this period worsens outcomes. With or without an operation, more than 80 percent of patients with obvious surgical indications eventually recover." [47]

But there are cases where back surgery may be necessary. I don't want chiropractors to appear to be as myopic as our medical counterparts who refuse to refer when indicated. My philosophy has always been to use the best of both worlds in health care so the patients benefit. But keep in mind that very few patients need back surgery and that this type of surgery often has very limited success rates. The AHCPR guideline recommends that if a patient doesn't respond to conservative care in an ample time frame (four to six weeks), then he or she should be referred for further testing.

First of all, just because you might be in a lot of pain, don't think surgery is the quick-fix solution. The guideline makes it quite clear that you shouldn't rush into surgery because of intense acute pain. For many patients, pain is the great motivator, especially when a surgeon convinces them that surgery is the quick answer to their back pain. Again, follow the guideline which advises patients to use acetaminophen or NSAIDs, ice/heat, and spinal manipulation for the first month. Then if nothing improves, explore the surgical route. Just remember: Back surgery may give some patients relief, but surgery doesn't stabilize their deconditioned spines. Consequently, more surgery often follows in an attempt to resolve future problems. Just as bypass heart surgery doesn't cure heart disease, unless significant life style changes are instituted by the patient, another heart surgery usually occurs every three or four years. Indeed, while back surgery may appear to be a quick-fix, it certainly isn't a total cure solving your bad back.

Again, let Dr. Ruth Jackson summarize the true indications for cervical fusion:

"Surgical operations on the cervical spine should not be undertaken lightly, and there should be very definite and positive indications for such procedures before they are contemplated. Inter-scapular pain is not sufficient reason for disc removal and inter-body fusion by the anterior approach, nor is a small amount of ligamentous instability sufficient indication for fusion. When, then, should fusion be done? Certain fracture-dislocations with marked instability may need fusion. Marked ligamentous instability with spinal cord irritation, or if there is danger of cord involvement, may indicate the necessity for fusion.

"...Surgery should be avoided unless there are absolute and definite indications for it, otherwise the results from operative procedures will be disappointing and the symptoms may be worse than they were before surgery was done. These cases are treatment cases which require time, patience and understanding, but the results will be gratifying." [48]

Dr. Jackson omitted in her surgical recommendations the most common diagnoses of "slipped disc" or "ruptured disc" or "degenerated disc" or "bone spurs," the most commonly given indications for back surgery by most surgeons. As Dr. Jackson writes, there are actually very few positive indications and they generally involve rare and serious spinal cord irritation: "The importance of cervical investigation in any patient with head, neck chest, shoulder and arm pain cannot be overemphasized. The usual diagnosis of arthritis, bursitis, neuritis, muscular rheumatism, fibrositis, fasciitis, tendinitis, pseudo-angina, migraine, etc. should not be made until cervical nerve root irritation has been ruled out entirely, if that is possible – which it usually is." [49]

But what if you have tried chiropractic care for one month and you still have the intense sciatic leg pain or back pain? If you've given conservative care adequate time and you've done your homework exercises and been a good patient, generally speaking, then you may be that one in 200 cases that needs further testing. Red flags for physiologic dysfunction include neurologic dysfunction, infection, inflammation, malignancy or other systemic illnesses. Other tests may look for anatomical reasons for the pain, such as a true ruptured disc, spinal stenosis, infection, tumor or abdominal mass causing referred pain. Again, these tests should only be done after at least one month of conservative care if no improvement whatsoever is achieved.

Let me quote from the AHCPR guideline on the different tests and treatments for these exceptional cases.[49]

"Special Studies: Tests for Evidence of Physiologic Dysfunction
Electrophysiologic Tests (EMG and SEP)

1. Needle EMG and H-reflex tests of the lower limb may be useful in assessing questionable nerve root dysfunction in patients with leg symptoms lasting longer than four weeks (regardless of whether patients also have back pain).

2. Surface EMG and F-wave tests are not recommended for assessing patients with low back symptoms.

3. SEPs may be useful in assessing suspected spinal stenosis and spinal cord myelopathy.

4. Bone Scan is recommended to evaluate acute low back problems when spinal tumor, infection or occult fracture is suspected from "red flags" on medical history, physical examination or collaborative lab test or plain x-ray findings.

5. Thermography is not recommended for assessing patients with acute low back problems.

"Special Studies: Tests to Provide Anatomic Definition

"In addition to x-rays, the imaging studies most generally used to define a possible anatomic cause for evidence of physiologic abnormalities include plain myelography, MRI, CT, CT-myelography, discography and CT-discography.

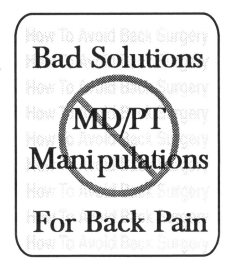

"Abnormal findings on anatomic studies such as MRI, CT, myelography, and discography may be misleading, however, if they are not corroborated with evidence of physiologic abnormality from the medical history, physical examination or physiologic tests. One problem with imaging studies is that in many patients, there is an inability to find any defects. Another problem is the lack of a "gold standard" in determining if an anatomic defect seen on imaging tests is actually the cause of symptoms. Anatomic abnormalities of the lumbar spine, such as degenerative changes and bulging or herniated discs, are found to increase with aging on x-rays and other imaging tests in subjects asymptomatic for low back problems.

"Several studies stress the importance of not relying too heavily on imaging studies alone for assessment when nerve root compromise is suspected. The anatomic level of imaging study findings must correspond to the side and the level of concern physiologically detected through the history, physical examination or other physiologic methods.

"Degenerative discs, bulging discs and even herniated discs are part of the aging process for the spine and may be irrelevant findings; they are seen on imaging tests of the lumbar spine in a significant percentage of subjects with no history of low back problems. Therefore, abnormal imaging findings seen in a patient with acute low back problems may or may not be related to that individual's symptoms.

"Surgery for Herniated Disc: Panel Recommendations

1. It is recommended that the treating clinician discuss further treatment options with the patient with sciatica after approximately one month of

conservative therapy. The clinician should consider referral to a specialist when all of the following conditions are met: (1) sciatica is both severe and disabling; (2) symptoms of sciatica persist without improvement or with progression; and (3) there is clinical evidence of nerve root compromise.

2. Patients with acute low back pain alone, who have neither suspicious findings for a significant nerve root compression nor any positive "red flags," do not need surgical consultation for possible herniated lumbar disc.

3. Reported complications of herniated disc surgery include operative mortality, wound infection, discitis, dural tears, nerve root injuries, thrombophlebitis and pulmonary emboli, meningitis, cauda equina syndrome, psoas hematoma, vascular injuries and risks associated with transfusions.

4. In the absence of fracture, dislocation or complications of tumor or infection, the use of spinal fusion is not recommended for the treatment of low back problems during the first three months of symptoms. Spinal fusion should be considered following decompression at a level of increased motion due to degenerative spondylolisthesis. There appears to be no good evidence from controlled trails that spinal fusion alone is effective for treatment of any type of acute low back problems in the absence of spinal fracture or dislocations... Moreover, there is no good evidence that patients who undergo fusion will return to their prior functional level."

As you can read for yourself, the actual cases that may need back surgery are few and far between. Moreover, recently the president of the International Society for the Study of the Lumbar Spine, Juergen Kraemer, MD, reported in *Spine* that "only 0.25 percent of individuals with back problems require surgery. Conservative care is the option of choice, which has been known by chiropractors for 100 years. All efforts must be made to prevent the worst course and prognosis of disc disease – the iatrogenic spine (failed back surgery syndrome)." When Dr. Kraemer presented his summary to that German orthopedic society, he concluded, "If you still love your patient with discogenic sciatica who gets tired of your conservative treatments, send him to a clinic with a long waiting list."[50] Better yet, send them to another chiropractor!

Keep in mind that intense back pain alone seldom requires surgery. Don't be mislead by some surgeon who exploits your situation by promising to resolve your pain instantly with a back surgery. On the other hand, if you are experiencing the "red flags" associated with back pain – infection, weight loss, fracture, trauma, neurological dysfunction – then further special studies are appropriate. But these occur in very few cases – one in 200 according to the panel of experts. Follow the recommendations of the AHCPR and in the long run, you'll be glad you did.

Remember what Dr. Robert Mendelsohn said: "Anyone who has a back surgery without seeing a chiropractor first should also have his head examined." Considering the recommendations of this panel of experts, I dare say that anyone who ignores its advice and has a back surgery without following its guideline should have his or her head examined! Back surgery is no minor issue, and since it is considered by the experts to be helpful in only one in 100 cases, it should be used only as a risky, last resort. Follow the advice of Dr. Mendelsohn and the AHCPR experts and seek conservative, chiropractic care first for your back pain problems.

Failed Back Surgery Syndrome

Unfortunately, many patients haven't followed this sage advice and have undergone back surgeries. Whether they just didn't know about the new recommendations of better options to their back pain problems, or they were misguided by their surgeon's *voo-doo* recommendation, or perhaps some never considered chiropractic care due to historical prejudice – for whatever reasons – too many people fall victim to these unnecessary, ineffective and expensive surgeries. And this tragedy hasn't slowed despite the overwhelming research and new federal guideline on acute low back pain, leaving an ever increasing wake of destruction in its path.

Actually, the insurance industry has created a separate billing code for such cases titled "failed back surgery syndrome." Since the AHCPR guideline on acute low back pain mentions that only one percent of back surgeries is helpful, this implies that 99 percent are considered not helpful, which means a lot of people are still suffering after their surgeries. The panel also found that 5 percent of low back patients accounts for 60 percent of the costs, principally these victims of unnecessary and ineffective back surgeries. In fact, who doesn't know someone who has had a failed back surgery and still suffers? Unfortunately, too many of us know of family or friends who were mislead by false hopes and misinformation into this epidemic.

But what if you've already had a back surgery? This is a predicament which thousands upon thousands of people face in this country every year. So, what are these failed back surgery patients to do? If they've been victimized by the *voo-doo* diagnosis designed to scare them about chiropractic care, they rarely think of it as a possible solution. Instead, these poor victims are fearful that adjustments

<figure>
To Avoid
Back Pain &
Spinal Surgery

Chiropractic

Exercise

Medical Box
Drugs
Hospitalizations
Surgeries

Weight Loss

Posture

The solution is
to think out of
the box!
</figure>

might leave them worse off than ever! *"You can't touch me with a 10-foot pole,"* is a comment I hear all too often from these medical failures. For these misinformed and scared people, chiropractic is not the "last resort," it is a "no resort" because they just don't think chiropractic care can help them now.

The fact is just the opposite. I've adjusted patients with discectomies, fusions, laminectomies and some with pedicle screws and plates in their spines. Keep in mind that chiropractors adjust spinal joints, not the discs themselves, so the adjustments are very safe and effective. Plus, we adjust areas above and below the points of surgery that become painful afterward, since the spine is still misaligned and unstable. Even if you've had spinal surgery, the chances are you can still be helped by chiropractic care. For the worst cases, many non-forceful methods of spinal adjusting are available as well that will stabilize your spinal weakness without any force or pain whatsoever.

Most patients with failed surgeries improve with chiropractic care, although their recovery is slower than with non-operative patients. I've found that these deconditioned patients not only are still full of spinal joint misalignments (the real cause of their back pain), but now their musculature is even weaker than before their surgery. Recreating spinal stability is a tough, uphill road for these patients, but they do improve as long as they follow a simple program of spinal adjustments and exercises.

The reason these patients still hurt after their spinal surgeries is because their spinal joints are still subluxated. At best, the disc surgery might relieve the herniation pressure upon the nerve root, but it does not realign their spinal joints and restore proper joint play. Nor does the surgery strengthen their spinal musculature. All these surgeries do is address the secondary problems of disc abnormalities or bone spurs. In fact, these post-operative patients are still misaligned, more deconditioned, and now suffer from the side-effects of surgery and debilitating bed rest causing joint fibrosis/stiffness and loss of muscular strength. And they wonder why they're not feeling any better. Again, just as bypass heart surgery is a band-aid solution, so are most back surgeries.

Although some of these medical failures are scared that an adjustment might "break loose" their fusions, there is no evidence of that occurring. Actually what does occur after a fusion is increased instability above and below the fusion, leading to more back pain and often times, additional surgeries. That's how the medical con game continues: "Another disc has herniated and needs to be removed." If you understand that the surgery did nothing to re-create spinal alignment, this will explain why patients still feel terrible and how patients are seduced into more surgeries. To stop this downward spiral of more back pain and additional back surgery, you need to learn how the spine actually works and why spinal manipulation can still help these cases. The more you learn about spinal mechanics, the more you will understand that the surgery does absolutely nothing to correct the fundamental underlying cause of your back pain – the vertebral subluxation.

Don't be surprised after you start feeling better under chiropractic care if you hear yourself asking, "Why didn't the MD send me to a chiropractor first?" I love to hear this question, although I realize it comes with a heavy price and after a lot of suffering. It's definitely no fun for patients to realize they've been lied to about chiropractic, and exploited and impaired by their MDs. For example, a young woman came to see me after two cervical fusions with metal plates and pedicle screws imbedded in her neck. Apparently, she simply awoke one morning with numbness in both arms and a severe headache. Two cervical surgeries and over $57,000 later, she still hurt just as badly and came to see me as the "last resort." Meanwhile, her MD learned of her dissatisfaction and ordered her to have another myelogram to determine if she needed a third surgery. When the myelogram came back negative, her surgeon told her that apparently her neck problem wasn't caused by a disc herniation and implied that her pain was all in her head! The fact is that her problems actually stemmed from an Atlas/Axis subluxation which caused spinal cord facilitation and nerve root pressure. Do you think she was mad when she improved with chiropractic adjustments and realized she never needed two neck surgeries?

Don't let this scenario happen to you. If it already has and you're a victim of a failed back surgery, now is the time to think out of the "medical box" of solutions. It's never too late to learn there is a better, safer, cheaper and more effective way to salvage this terrible situation without enduring another unnecessary surgery or living a life in pain. Even though these victims of failed surgeries possibly have been taught by their surgeons to be fearful of spinal adjustments, until they are adjusted, their back pain will never improve. (The irony of such misinformation is beyond comprehension – to think an adjustment is more dangerous than spinal surgery – perhaps Dr. Mendelsohn was right to state that anyone who has a back surgery first should have his head examined!)

In the next chapter I will explain the logic and science of chiropractic spinal care. Then you can understand how this care will help anyone overcome back pain and avoid another disabling surgery, even those victims of failed back surgery.

CHAPTER FOUR

The Clinical Practice of Chiropractic

*"You know you're getting old
when your back goes out
more often than you do!"*
– Bob Hope, American comedian

Ⅎ love giving patients a good spinal adjustment. Beforehand, I can see the pain in their eyes and I can feel the spastic muscles and joint stiffness in their spines. Afterward, I can see in the patients' faces the immediate relief that comes from a good adjustment. I can sense the relief from pain in their spinal joints when the adjustments make that wonderful popping noise that tells me the joint play is restored. When I feel their spinal joints move, I know that patients will soon begin to feel better. And, as a patient myself, I love getting adjustments. My three chronic spinal injuries need regular maintenance care, and only spinal adjustments have helped me from living a life in pain. Actually, if it wasn't for chiropractic care, I wouldn't be able to do my job as a chiropractor, because adjusting patients is probably one of the most physically challenging treatments to render in the health-care world. Indeed, it's tough being a chiropractor in many ways, but all the obstacles and difficulties are worth the emotional and professional tribulations because there's absolutely no substitute in the entire medical world for a good spinal adjustment.

The first adjustment is my favorite one to give. Most patients are totally unaware of a traditional chiropractic adjustment, and are inherently worried about any treatment, are fearful of medical *voo-doo* stories about chiropractic care, and generally are quite apprehensive. I admire their courage to overcome these fears and submit themselves to a treatment unlike anything they've ever experienced before. Some people are relaxed, but most have sweaty palms when they lie down on the adjusting table for the first time. Actually, sometimes I wish I could have a candid video camcorder in my adjusting room to record the funny reactions patients have during their first adjustment. Rarely before have they had a doctor literally wrestle with them and never before have they heard their spines go "pop." I enjoy watching their eyes widen when they feel and hear their spinal joints release for the very first time. Afterwards, I love to hear them say, *"That didn't feel bad at all, actually it felt good."*

In fact, a good chiropractic adjustment feels great! At that moment, the patients' fears, worries and concerns vanish when they experience the relief from their very first adjustment. Only then do they realize that the medical horror stories were bunk and their years of suffering will soon be over. Some patients, especially those victims of failed back surgery, become angry and flatly state,

"Why didn't my MD tell me the truth and send me to a chiropractor first?" Other patients give a sigh of relief as they rest on the adjusting table when they experience the release of pressure on their joints and nerves. Some immediately tell me, *"Now I understand why my friends tell me chiropractic care can be addictive because it feels so good."* The satisfaction from the first adjustment is an experience to behold, but only chiropractors have the rare opportunity to share this moment with their patients.

Once patients experience their initial series of spinal adjustments, a remarkable change of attitude generally occurs. At first, patients are hurting, skeptical and quite upset about being a medical failure. They're still in pain despite their medications, hot packs, physical therapy and back surgeries. They're tired of being disabled by their back pain, they're upset about spending a lot of money on failed medical treatments and they're unsure about going to a chiropractic clinic because of their medical brainwashing they received through the years. Nonetheless, despite all these negatives, after their first few adjustments, most patients are quite satisfied with their decision to go to a chiropractor. Then the change of attitude happens – frowning, skeptical people become smiling patients, happy to be coming for their adjustments. Ignorant, skeptical attitudes become grateful and appreciative when patients learn the truth about spinal care. And most of all, a greater appreciation occurs when they learn that you don't need just a backache to see a chiropractor.

The transformation from a medical skeptic into a successful and satisfied chiropractic patient is the most rewarding of all experiences for chiropractors. We know that spinal adjustments will help the majority of back problems, but when patients learn and understand the logic and science of chiropractic care, then we've accomplished a much more important task. We've opened the door out of their medical boxed-in thinking for the first time in their lives. We've liberated them from a life of drugs and unnecessary surgeries. We've given them a new understanding about health and given them a new avenue to better health, naturally. Indeed, going to a chiropractor is a radical act that transcends simply giving patients another treatment option for their back pain. It is very much a consciousness-raising experience. Indeed, it is a Renaissance of health care for many people.

But many unaware people have neither experienced chiropractic adjustments nor understood chiropractic's logic of spinal health. And, before they will understand, many questions must be answered, such as: *"What do chiropractors actually do?"*, *"Are adjustments safe?"*, *"What's a typical treatment plan,"* and most importantly, *"What do I have to do to keep my spine healthy, pain-free and to avoid a relapse?"*

Let's talk about the "hows" and "whys" of this misunderstood profession. Let's overcome your skepticism with a realistic description of the clinical practice of a chiropractor. In fact, in order for it to have the greatest possible impact in their lives, I prefer my patients to *understand* chiropractic care and not just to *believe* in it.

Most patients never get a clear picture of chiropractic until they actually visit a chiropractic office. Even then, not all DCs take the time to teach their patients as they treat them. Few DCs give health classes or back schools to explain the logic and science of chiropractic care; instead they focus principally on the treatment plans. Consequently, many satisfied patients remain uninformed about chiropractic science and while they may believe in chiropractic's effectiveness, they may not understand just know it works. Despite the fact that chiropractic celebrated its 100th birthday in 1995, most Americans still consider it to be a new health profession. Although it may seem new to them, in fact, the art of spinal manipulation is aged – going back to Hippocrates himself. But since it's probably new to you, let me explain the art and science of chiropractic and what may happen when you visit a chiropractor's office.

The Miraculous Spinal Column

I often think the public's misunderstanding about the source of most back pain stems from the misnomer of labeling the spine the "backbone." In fact, the spine should be called the "backbones" because it is comprised of numerous small bones called vertebrae that are interconnected by joints as well as discs. Instead of visualizing a singular bone, I suggest you instead think of a stack of small bones sitting atop one another, and then you may better understand the likelihood of misaligning this delicate pillar.

The spinal column has a unique design unlike any other part of your body. It is comprised of 24 vertebrae sitting on top of three pelvic bones, interconnected by 23 discs and 137 spinal joints, surrounded by six layers of ligaments and muscles. And on top of the spinal column sits your head, encasing the brain from which descends a spinal cord down through a canal in the spinal column. The spinal cord emits nerve roots which send bio-electrical "mental" impulses to energize every muscle, gland, organ and tissue cell in your body. The spinal column also is a weight-bearing skeletal system that supports your head, ribs, arms and torso. As you can see, your spinal column is a complex entity that is essential in many ways to your good health – if everything is working properly, that is.

Unfortunately, accidents happen. Whether it's a car accident, sports injury, a bicycle crash, a slip on wet pavement, lifting improperly or simply bad sitting and sleeping postures, there are many ways you can injure your spine. Although there may be different types of injury to your spine, by far <u>most spinal problems begin with the misalignment of the 137 joints that connect your spine.</u> When these spinal joints are misaligned, secondary problems also may occur such as torn ligaments, swollen discs, strain muscles and nerve pressure. Your back pain is actually a combination of all these potential sources of injury, and if there is also a "pinched nerve," additional pain will radiate down your arms or legs, causing radiating pain (sciatica) or will radiate into organs in your abdomen, causing organ malfunction as well as pain. But, for the most part, your back attack is mainly due to joint problems in your spine. That's why the ancient art of spinal manipulation of these joints has always been so effective in reducing back pain.

Before you can understand the objective of chiropractic care, you need to know what is considered the normal standard for a spine. It's rather simple actually – on the front view of your spinal column, your spine should be straight with a level pelvis that acts like the foundation of your entire spine. On the side view, your spine should have four curves which are essential for proper weight bearing and movement. The problem begins when you lose this normal geometric alignment of your spine. Then distortions, misalignments and vertebral subluxations happen, causing joint problems, a lack of joint play, nerve pressure, disc degeneration and scoliosis. The goal of our care is to restore as closely as possible the normal geometry and functioning of the spinal column. The closer to normal your spine becomes, the less likely it is that there will be joint dysfunction, nerve pressure and pain.

Of great importance in the rehabilitation of the spine is the nature of the major spinal joints. Unlike the hip joint which is a "ball and socket" type joint that is designed for weight-bearing, the spinal joints are not intended to bear weight. These joints are described as "gliding" joints that interlock, but their movement primarily is to allow for flexion and rotation and not for bearing weight, like the hip joint. Obviously, in the animal kingdom vertebral animals walk on all four legs and use their spines as a beam. Only mankind has stood upright and used the spine as a post, causing these gliding joints to bear weight, and causing all the trouble. Instead

The Human Spinal Column

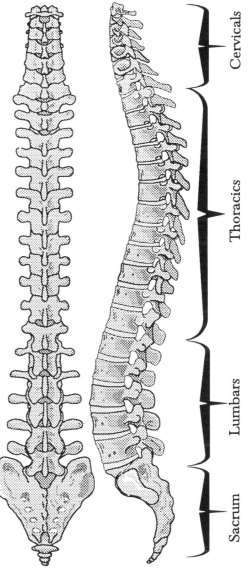

Cervicals

Thoracics

Lumbars

Sacrum

Back View **Side View**

of acting as a beam, the human spine acts as a pillar comprised of 24 building blocks that must balance a 12-pound head and bear the weight of our torso. Quite a feat, to say the least, and it leaves us very susceptible to injury, as well. This precarious column of bones, held together by six layers of ligaments and muscles is even more likely to misalign when traumatic forces enter the picture. Any accident, fall or sudden jerking movements can easily misalign the column of vertebrae, thus throwing the joints out of alignment and causing the soft tissues to become damaged.

There is another interesting and important point about the spine's design which explains why the majority of spinal misalignments occur at the very top and bottom of the spine. As I stated, there are 23 intervertebral discs that act as shock-absorbers between each vertebrae, except for the very top one called the Atlas. Just as the Greek god Atlas held up the Earth, so too does this vertebral Atlas hold up the skull. Unfortunately, this donut-shaped vertebrae has no disc between it and the head or the second vertebrae beneath it, named the Axis. Without disc cartilage to cushion and hold the vertebrae firmly in place, this Atlas easily can misalign and cause a multitude of problems, both in terms of spinal mechanics

and neurological problems, because the brain stem resides in this area of the spinal cord. Obviously any misalignment in this upper cervical area may cause severe joint restrictions – the typical stiff neck – but it also may cause severe headaches and nerve interference to the major organs. In fact, the top of your neck is, without question, the most important part of your spine to consider whenever there are health problems or headaches of any sort.

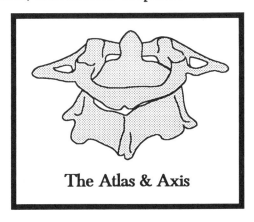

The Atlas & Axis

Another important area of the spine to consider, especially for low back pain, consists of the two sacroiliac joints in the pelvis. The 24 vertebrae sit atop the three bones of the pelvis – the sacrum (tailbone) and the two iliums (hip bones). These two sacroiliac joints bear the weight of your entire torso and are active in any movement. But again, these two joints are not ball and socket or even gliding joints as much as they simply "butt" up against each other without any disc, held together by ligaments and surrounded by layers of muscles. The vast majority of low back pain begins when one of these sacroiliac joints becomes misaligned, then the severe butt and leg pain – "sciatica" – begins.

Actually, in one study by J. L. Shaw, MD, this orthopedic investigator found that 98 percent of his patients with low back pain had sacroiliac misalignments as the primary cause. His research on 1,000 patients with low back and leg pain concluded that:

"98 percent of the patients had a mechanical dysfunction of the sacroiliac joints as the major cause of their low back pain...only two patients required disc surgery.
"The conventional wisdom is that herniated discs are responsible for low back pain, and that sacroiliac joints do not move significantly and do not cause low back pain or dysfunction. The ironic reality may well

be that sacroiliac joint dysfunctions are the major cause of low back dysfunction, as well as the primary factor causing disc space degeneration, and ultimate herniation of disc material."[1]

Once a sacroiliac joint misaligns, the entire lower back will compensate for it, causing more pain and problems in the lumbar spine. Too many back surgeries have been unsuccessful because this primary misalignment was ignored since there wasn't a disc to evaluate; instead the surgeons focus on the lumbar discs which may have herniated as a secondary response to the sacroiliac misalignment and the subsequent compensatory spinal distortion.

It is crucial to examine these two areas of your spine if you have any hope of stabilizing your spinal column. Considering the precarious nature of the spine itself – 24 small bones held together by small ligaments and muscles, balanced precariously by 137 non-weight bearing joints – you can understand how difficult it is to repair this spinal column when injury strikes. No matter where your pain or problems may be, I suggest you have your entire spine evaluated to determine how it functions overall, because any misalignment at the top or bottom will cause the rest of the spine to compensate, setting the stage for scoliosis and distortions to develop elsewhere. Even though the spine is comprised of numerous vertebrae sitting atop three pelvic bones interconnected by a multitude of joints, it acts as one unit. So, even if you're experiencing pain at one end of your spine, the structural cause may actually originate at the other end. Only a thorough chiropractic analysis will determine the geometry of your spine and the likelihood of future spinal problems.

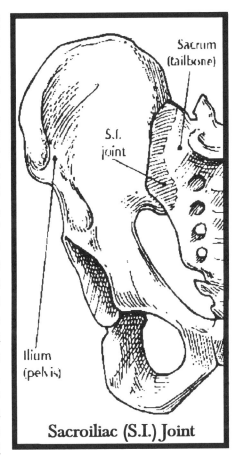

Sacroiliac (S.I.) Joint

After years of instability and misalignments, the spine begins to deteriorate and spinal arthritis develops – disc degeneration, bone spurs, joint arthritis and nerve damage. Just as your teeth degenerate if neglected, so will your spine. But these secondary consequences are not the cause of most back pain; they are simply effects of the underlying misalignments, and treating them with surgery never helps. Until the mechanical problem (the lack of proper alignment and joint play) is corrected, no spine will work well or without pain. Perhaps now you can understand why back surgery fails in the majority of cases when surgeons ignore the joint issue and focus solely on the secondary problems with discs. Obviously, it's easier to understand that back pain caused by spinal joint dysfunction is a serious problem that requires more than simply pain pills or muscle relaxants and less treatment than back surgery. Now that you understand the functioning of the 137 joints in the spine, it is easier to see why spinal manipulation works so well.

The Vertebral Subluxation Complex

I would estimate that 90 percent of new patients have no idea what chiropractors do or how we do it, probably because there's never been a chiropractor on a television sitcom or news stories showing the public our professional treatments. So let me explain exactly what a vertebral subluxation is, what an adjustment does and the nature of spinal care. All these are good questions which need to be answered before you can make an informed decision about seeking chiropractic care.

Let's take a close look at what happens when you injure your spinal column. Aside from the very few serious fractures, cancers or other pathologies which require medical care, most spinal problems stem from the misalignment of your spinal vertebrae – the *vertebral subluxation* as we chiropractors refer to these injuries. Vertebrae are the 24 small bones in the spinal column and subluxation simply means a slight misalignment. There are five major components of a vertebral subluxation complex, and the repair of your back problem will depend on how well each of these factors is handled.

Most people with back problems have stiffness in their spinal joints. This first component is called *kinesiopathology*, which means abnormal movement or motion in the spinal joints. Too little movement is called *hypomobility*, which we chiropractors term *fixations* and our patients simply call stiffness. Too much movement is called *hypermobility*, which happens in whiplash-type situations when the ligaments or muscles are strained and allow excessive joint play. Another type of abnormal movement develops when a long-standing misalignment from childhood develops into scoliosis curves elsewhere in the spine. This is called a *compensatory reaction* and unfortunately is seen in many adults who never had their spines adjusted as children after everyday accidents on playgrounds.

Once a misalignment occurs, causing abnormal movement in the spinal joints, the second component of nerve interference may follow – the *pinched nerve* as most people call it. Let me first explain that not every spinal misalignment is considered a *vertebral subluxation*, because there are technical differences between the two. While both are structural abnormalities that appear out of normal alignment with the vertebrae above or below, vertebral subluxation is more serious since it causes nerve interference as well as joint pain. Patients may have many spinal misalignments but only a few true vertebral subluxations causing nerve interference. In other words, spinal injuries may cause joint problems and back pain, but until these misalignments cause nerve interference, they are not technically called vertebral subluxations. While this difference may seem minor, it actually is the difference between just a back pain and dysfunction in organs or muscles.

When a misalignment causes the pinched nerve syndrome, this is technically called *neuropathophysiology* – a malfunction of the nerve system resulting from the misalignment of the spinal vertebrae. The shooting pains or numbness down your arms or legs is a good example of this component. Aside from the classic pinched nerve (pressure on nerve roots), malfunction of the nerve system may occur due to subluxation by stretching or twisting of the spinal cord itself. This type of nerve pressure is referred to as a *facilitative lesion.* Severe spinal distortions from scoliosis or birth trauma may cause the dura mater (the layers of skin covering the spinal cord) to swell or even bleed (hemorrhage). In a 1979 Harvard Medical School study on crib death (Sudden Infant Death Syndrome), conducted by Floyd Gilles, MD, forceps delivery was found in seven out of eight autopsies to be the cause of subdural hemorrhage in the neck.[2] In fact, subluxation of the top vertebrae in the neck can be a serious, if not a deadly matter for babies and for adults as well.

Like a game of dominoes, once the subluxation occurs the nerve pressure begins and muscle spasm follows. This third component is called *myopathology*, which simply means that your muscles aren't working right because of the pinched nerve syndrome. Symptoms may include spasms, loss of strength or muscle balance, swelling, inflammation or edema. Flaccid paralysis will occur if the nerve pressure continues and is not corrected. That's why patients with pinched nerves who are not adjusted see their muscle tone change from spasm to flaccidity – from too much tone to too little tone. Most patients understand that pinched nerves can cause muscle spasms in their arms or legs, but few realize that the same process of muscle spasm may lead to more serious conditions such as hypertension or asthma.

Changes also occur in the ligaments and disc cartilage either by being stretched or torn. These problems are termed *histopathology*, which means abnormalities in the tissues around the spinal column. Disc swelling or herniation results only after the subluxation has occurred, and if uncorrected, in time the disc swelling will proceed to disc degeneration or possible rupture. But the thing to remember is that no disc becomes abnormal until a misalignment occurs first. The disc is secondary at all times to the spinal misalignment in the course of degeneration – no disc degenerates because it wants to; it only does so when it's forced to by the misaligned vertebrae. Never forget this vital point.

The area of the vertebral subluxation complex best known by the public is the arthritic component called *pathophysiology.* Again, using the domino effect, after a spine becomes misaligned, it actually is weakened as a weight-bearing column. To strengthen these weak areas, the body sends calcium salts to the vertebrae, resulting in bone spurs on the vertebrae. While this may help to shore up a weakened area, it may also cause nerve pressure as well. This double-edge sword is a result of the initial subluxation and can be prevented if adjusted in time. In addition, calcium is deposited in the joints, causing joint degeneration and stiffness. This process of spinal arthritis is termed *subluxation degeneration*, and it occurs in most anyone who has never been to a chiropractor. As you can see, a vertebral subluxation is a dangerous situation that will not only cause intense pain, but which will lead to spinal arthritis and ill health as well.

Any hope to stopping back pain or the arthritic process of subluxation degeneration begins with the rehabilitation of your spine through chiropractic adjustments and spinal exercises. These components of the vertebral subluxation complex all will be improved when your spine has better joint alignment, muscular strength and joint flexibility. Restoring normal joint play and mobility is the cornerstone of the chiropractic adjustment. And proper muscular strength is essential to re-establishing spinal stability. When the vertebral subluxation misalignment is reduced by the adjustment and muscles are strengthened to *hold* the adjustment, then normal joint play will ensure a relief from nerve pressure, disc swelling and the other components that may lead to spinal degeneration. Only then will you feel better and stay better without back pain or spinal arthritis.

While this discussion of the five components of the vertebral subluxation complex may be more than the average person is interested in knowing, it does help you to understand the dynamics of these spinal problems. As you can see, the problems associated with this condition are more complex than simply a "slipped disc" or a "pulled muscle," as the MDs would tell you. And correcting these problems involves more than simply taking pain pills and muscle relaxants and less than having a dangerous, risky and expensive disc surgery. The more you understand about the five components of the vertebral subluxation complex, the better success you will have in the rehabilitation of your spine with the help of a chiropractor.

Spinal Joint Play

In solving the puzzle of back pain, the most important concept to keep in mind is that the spine is primarily a chain link of 24 vertebrae and three pelvic bones interconnected by 137 joints. Forget about the disc concept – it is totally secondary in this puzzle of back pain. In this light, solving back pain and rehabilitating your spine is actually a matter of restoring the normal function of the many joints in your spinal column. When any joint has proper alignment, strength and flexibility, then it will move and function normally and without pain, stiffness or weakness – a concept referred to as *joint play*.

Most back pain is simply the loss of normal joint play. And the primary aim of a spinal adjustment is to restore the normal joint play of your spinal joints. It's when your spinal joints lose their normal joint play that stiffness, pain, disc and nerve pressure develops. Whether it's a fall that twists or jams your spinal joints together, a whiplash that tears the joints apart, or simply sitting too long and compressing your spinal joints, whenever your spinal joints lose their normal joint play, problems and pain arise.

It's very easy to lose the normal joint play in your spine considering the stresses we place on our backs every day. We ask our spines to withstand low-grade *micro*-traumatic events daily – sports, bending, lifting and twisting at work, aside from the occasional high-grade *macro*-traumas like accidents and falls that people experience. According to Dr. Richard Deyo, a leading researcher in this field, "The back is a complicated structure that we ask a lot of. You've got vertebrae, muscles, ligaments, nerve roots, the spinal cord, and a lot of weight stacked on, and you expect it to twist and bend in all directions."[3]

Compounding these traumatic events with a gradual deconditioned body that must endure constant, repetitive, passive stress like sitting for prolonged periods at computers, it's easy to understand why 80 percent of adults will have a back attack sometime in their lives. Considering the many traumas, constant stresses and occasional strains our spines encounter daily, it's little wonder why back attacks are epidemic and unavoidable. Now you can understand why your back "goes out" after years of traumas, stresses and strains! Indeed, as Bob Hope once joked, *"You know you're getting old when your back goes out more often than you do!"*

Dr. John McMillan Mennell, orthopedist, author, professor and a proponent of manipulation, testified at the chiropractic vs. AMA antitrust trial (*Wilk* case) about the nature of joint play, joint dysfunction, and manipulative therapy as the only solution to this epidemic problem:

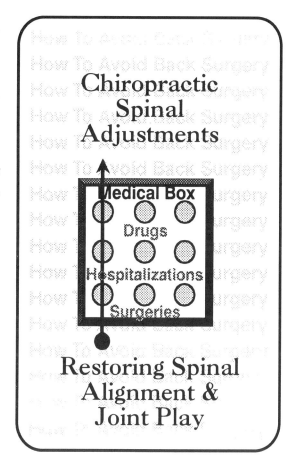

> "To understand it, you would have to accept that the science of mechanics demands that anything that moves has joint play built between the moving parts...This joint play movement, which is in everything that is made to move, is prerequisite to normal pain-free functioning of movement in that thing, whatever that thing may be.

> "...every joint has a synovial lining to it which 'secretes' fluid to maintain the viability of the joint... (in the spine there are) about 137 synovial joints between the lamina facets, the occipital condyles, the bottom of the skull as it rests on the atlas, the sacroiliac joints, the sacrococcygeal joints, even the joints of the fundusca in the neck...

> "...When you are dealing with manipulative therapy in the spine... your objective is to try to restore the proper motion joint play, which is

prerequisite to the normal function of the joint in the spine... the vertebra may be misaligned because of the loss of joint play in the synovial joints. So, the effect of the manipulation of the synovial joints is to realign the vertebra, but that is not the primary business...it's a result of it."[4]

Dr. Mennell mentioned during his testimony that 80 percent of patients who go to a family doctor complain about some form of musculoskeletal pain. He testified that:

"[E]ight out of 10 patients that come out of any doctor's office complain of a musculoskeletal system problem regardless of from what system the pain is coming... I will say 100 percent of those complaints, which are, in fact, due to joint dysfunction in the musculoskeletal system... I will say at some stage of recovery, there will be some local joint dysfunction in almost any patient....if you don't manipulate to relieve the symptoms from this condition of joint dysfunction, then you are depriving the patient of the one thing that is likely to relieve them of their suffering."[5]

This expert's testimony that spinal manipulation to correct joint dysfunction and to restore proper joint play is the only viable solution for these 80 percent of patients with back pain convinced a federal court judge that manipulation was an effective choice of treatment. Unfortunately, too many patients are being denied the one thing that can relieve them of their suffering – chiropractic spinal care. Dr. Mennell's testimony sheds light on a fact that has long been known by chiropractors: That the key to back pain problems is proper joint play in the 137 joints in the spine.

Spinal rehabilitation begins with restoring proper joint play. Your spinal health is not solely a function of your discs, as the medics would have you think. Your good spinal health is mostly a function of how well you maintain the proper joint play of the many joints between the vertebrae and three pelvic bones that comprise your spinal column.

Obviously, the purpose of a joint is to move properly, so if these spinal joints are misaligned due to trauma of any sort, the joint dysfunction may lead to back pain, pinched nerves, joint stiffness, as well as degeneration and spinal curvature later in life. It all starts with the initial spinal joint misalignments causing the loss of normal joint play. The goal of chiropractic adjustments is to restore the normal joint play – the alignment and flexibility of the misalignments in your spine. Spinal exercises are aimed at increasing muscular strength and flexibility in order to maintain normal joint play. The answer to the question *"Why does manipulation work so well?"* is easy to understand when you recognize joint play as the key to a healthy, functioning, pain-free spine.

You can be the strongest person in the world, but if your spine is subluxated you will be in a great deal of pain. And if these subluxations remain uncorrected, a permanent distortion will develop and lead to spinal pathologies like disc degeneration and bone spurs. Only chiropractic adjustments can correct these misaligned, subluxated joints by restoring normal joint play and, thereby, relieve joint pain and nerve pressure. Keep your spinal joints aligned and flexible, your spinal muscles strong, and you'll experience the best possible spinal health.

The Chiropractic Adjustment

Now that you have a general understanding of the anatomy of the spine and the importance of normal joint play, the next question is, *"How do we actually help patients?"*

MDs have their drugs and scalpels, dentists have their drills, and chiropractors have their hands to render spinal adjustments. Actually, the word "chiropractic" is of Greek origin and means "to practice by hands." Although DCs utilize many types of equipment and instruments to help restore spinal function, traditional chiropractic care consists of adjusting the spinal column joints manually with the hands to correct vertebral subluxations.

The chiropractic adjustment is a wonderful act that is sadly unknown to the public. Most people have heard that chiropractors "crack" or "pop" the back, but we prefer not to use those terms, because they imply fractures or pain – similar to saying "salmonella" in a restaurant. Although the adjustment of the spinal joints may make the same type of noise as when you "pop" your knuckles, it is merely a locked joint able to freely move again, and the popping noise is caused by the release of gas in the fixated joint itself. The technical term for this audible sound is *joint cavitation*, and it is painless in and of itself. In other words, joint manipulation does not hurt, but if the patient has damaged soft tissues around the joint, the manipulation may aggravate the swollen and tender tissues, similar to adjusting a sprained ankle.

There is no bone breaking or cracking when you hear the popping noise during an adjustment. It is merely the sound of a joint that is misaligned and stiff becoming more flexible again. That's why patients feel an immediate relief after an adjustment, because they can feel the freedom of movement. And since there are numerous sensory nerves in the joint itself, an adjustment relieves pressure upon these nerves, as well as pressure on the nerve root and disc. But please don't tell others that a chiropractor "cracks" your back, because that might scare them away and deny them the myriad of benefits associated with this spinal care.

The chiropractic adjustment itself simple takes a joint beyond its normal physiological range of motion but not past its anatomical range of motion. In simple terms, this means that when a joint becomes misaligned, it automatically loses its normal range of motion – the normal joint play. In most cases, especially long-standing chronic cases, the spinal joints become hypomobile, meaning that they lose their range of motion and become stiff. In some traumatic cases like a whiplash, the joints initially become hypermobile – they are too loose and highly unstable. If a joint is hypomobile and has lost its normal range of motion, an adjustment will be aimed at increasing the joint play. If a joint is hypermobile, the adjustment will be aimed at realignment to decrease the excessive joint play, and spinal exercises will help to stabilize the joint. The goal of chiropractic care is to stabilize the weakened spinal area with corrective spinal adjustments and to strengthen the muscles with spinal exercises, thus restoring normal joint play.

The Nature of Spinal Care

Before any patient receives treatment from a DC, a thorough spinal exam is conducted. It includes an x-ray of the spine to determine the spinal distortions and any pathologies, a spinal physical exam to determine the movement and functioning of the spine, and in some traumatic cases, a spinal muscle test is performed to determine the relative strength of the spine. These exams reveal the alignment, strength and flexibility of the spine – the three basic principles of spinal rehabilitation.

The spinal x-ray analysis and spinal physical exam give an overall picture of your spinal distortions, also known as scoliosis, and of specific vertebral subluxations or individual spinal misalignments causing nerve pressure and joint pain. Ironically, not every spinal distortion is the source of either back pain or nerve pressure. I have seen patients whose x-rays revealed severe scoliosis, but who had only minor back pain because their spinal joints were flexible. On the other hand, I've seen patients with what appeared to be good spinal x-rays with few misalignments who were in severe pain because they had lost their normal joint movement. The key to whether or not a spine is painful primarily rests on the amount of joint play in the spinal joints. Again, all three principles – alignment, strength and flexibility – determine how well a spine functions, and all three must be taken into account in an analysis of your spinal integrity.

Before any treatment plan begins, a thorough report is given to the patient to review the tests results and to explain the nature of the treatment plan itself. This is important, because too often patients think their spinal problem is a minor problem and that the treatment should be a one-time event – like *"pulling a thorn out of a paw."* Wrong. Most spinal problems take years to create. A treatment plan is not unlike a rehab program for an injured football player. Spinal rehab is not a one-time treatment; it is a slow process that takes time and effort.

How much time it will take to feel better is a main concern for most patients. The new U.S. Public Health Service guideline on acute low back pain suggests at least four weeks of conservative care for pain control to determine whether or not spinal manipulation will be effective. If no improvement is noted in that time frame, the guideline suggests referral for more extensive testing. I have found that most patients feel better after two to four weeks of intensive care, with adjustments and ice therapy or electro-therapy in the most severe cases. Although the first goal of care (pain control) may come within a few weeks, don't be fooled into thinking that your spine is "cured" forever just because the pain has lessened. The second goal of chiropractic treatment is to stabilize the weakened spinal area to avoid a possible relapse. Believe me when I tell you that a relapse will likely happen if rehabilitative and maintenance care are not emphasized.

Basically, a standard chiropractic treatment plan consists of three types of care. Intensive care is aimed at controlling pain, and during this two to four week period the patient may be seen daily and given spinal adjustments and therapy to reduce the pain and swelling. Rehabilitative care begins once the pain is under control, with the goal of stabilizing the spinal weakness. Patients are given spinal conditioning exercises and weekly adjustments aimed at correcting the major spinal subluxations. Rehabilitative care continues on average from one to four months, or longer if the patient is overweight or extremely out of shape. Once the patient has reached the point of maximum correction, maintenance care is recommended at least monthly in order to preserve the correction. Daily home spinal exercises and monthly maintenance care is essential to avoid a relapse. This is a hard concept for many patients to understand, but those who do subscribe to this notion have the longest lasting results. Indeed, an ounce of prevention is worth a pound of cure!

Although a chiropractor can adjust the many spinal joints to restore joint play and to relieve your back pain, you shouldn't assume that your pain is gone forever. The dynamics of the spine – the functioning of the numerous joints between the bony segments of the spinal column – makes for a very tenuous situation. Considering the many forces, stresses, loads and bad leverages we place on our spines daily, you cannot assume that one or two chiropractic adjustments will cure you of back pain for the rest of your life. Let's talk about stabilizing your spine instead of just controlling pain. Let's focus on reconditioning your entire body to help maintain your spinal integrity and to avoid a relapse and eventual spinal degeneration.

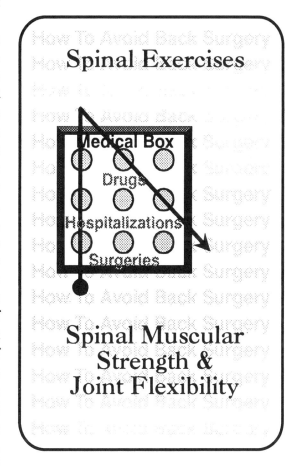

After the initial spinal treatment plan is finished, I always conduct a re-examination to see what is left to treat. As I tell my patients, the initial exam reveals the starting point. Their permanent spinal pattern cannot be determined until they've been through the treatment plan. After a series of adjustments and with time for the spinal exercises to become effective, a re-exam then will determine their final spinal status. Whatever is left is considered their point of maximum improvement and must be maintained, or it will worsen and a relapse is quite possible. The patient's "Progress Report" is a most interesting consultation, since it shows the impact of the adjustments and exercises. If the patient has been dutiful and cooperative in his or her treatment plan, the back pain or nerve interference will be gone and the alignment, strength and flexibility may improve. If the patient has been negligent in his or her exercises, while the pain may have improved, the most important factors may not have improved. Whatever is left at the "Progress Report" mostly likely is their permanent pattern that must be maintained or else the correction may be lost, may worsen and relapse again.

Maintenance spinal care is a difficult concept for many patients. Whereas most people give proactive care to their teeth, few people are proactive about their spines. Too often satisfied patients who complete their initial treatment plan mistakenly think they're "cured for life" and fail to maintain their correction, only to experience a relapse later. Forget about pain as your only criteria for back care – it's similar to brushing your teeth only when they hurt! We know that's a silly notion, but too often spinal patients forget to maintain their spinal correction with daily spinal exercises and periodic spinal check-ups. Maintenance spinal care is as important if not more important to your overall health than dental care. That's why in my office we teach our patients to develop a *"dental attitude"* towards their spines.

Some people unaware of the need for continued care may perceive ongoing care as unnecessary. Too often I've heard the rap against maintenance care by the uninformed: *"If you go to a chiropractor, you have to go the rest of your life."* My response is simply, *"You'll go to the dentist the rest of your life, so what's the problem with the concept of maintenance spinal care?"*

The problem is that most people are unaccustomed to daily spinal exercises and monthly chiropractic adjustments as a necessary routine. The transition from being an acute patient to a proactive, maintenance care patient is a quantum leap for many people. While some get this idea, many people only use chiropractic care as 911 emergency care when they suffer a relapse. Unfortunately, some patients just don't learn there's a better way to approach their health needs than merely chasing symptoms and pain with quick-fix solutions.

The Importance of Spinal Exercises

Too often some patients mistakenly rely completely upon spinal adjustments for spinal health. Without daily spinal exercises to restore spinal muscle strength and joint play, the spines cannot stabilize. And as you gracefully age, your spinal muscles become weaker and the possibility of relapse is more likely. It is imperative to do daily spinal exercises – the equivalent of "toothpaste" in the maintenance of your spinal health-care. If you don't do them regularly, when your spine does relapse, you'll have only yourself to blame.

Daily spinal exercises will strengthen weak spinal muscles that have been damaged by trauma or weakened from years of neglect, and will help you to hold the adjustment for longer periods. Failure to strengthen these six layers of spinal muscles will only add to your back problems, because subluxations will occur more often causing the regrettable relapse and progressive degeneration.

According to Burl Pettibone, DC, a leading chiropractic clinical technique developer, "The patient must understand that most subluxation complexes are not merely 'bones out of place', but also altered physiology and pathology

78

changes of their paravertebral supportive structure soft tissue. These must be arrested, reversed and rehabilitated before the correction can be expected to be maintained." [6]

Spinal exercises are based upon spinal mechanics and spinal physiology and are necessary to maintain proper strength, flexibility and nourishment to the muscles, joints, discs and ligaments of the spine. After age 25, the spine undergoes physiological changes, namely, decreased blood supply to the discs and ligaments. Nourishment to the discs then occurs only when the spine undergoes full range of motion exercises. Although the disc no longer has whole blood pumped around it, the ligaments are bathed in tissue cell fluid. This fluid has all the nutrients of whole blood and the ability to excrete waste products as well. The discs need the exercise motion to stimulate osmosis and inhibition with the intercellular fluids, thus keeping the disc properly nourished, lubricated and pliable.

The president of the International Society for the Study of the Lumbar Spine, Dr. Juergen Kraemer, reported in *Spine* magazine that the disc is an osmotic system that lives from motion. Because of our sedentary, non-moving, modern lifestyles, disc degeneration is progressive. Dr. Kraemer noted that "uptake of fluid into the disc takes place in lying and relaxed positions. Frequent changes of postures improve uptake, but high pressure postures, like sitting, inhibit disc nutrition." The progressive dehydration of disc material explains why few elderly people suffer from disc herniations, which are most common in mid-life. The average age of a disc surgery patient is only 42 years old. According to Dr. Kraemer, "In mid-life, we have the biomechanical constellation for disc herniations – the nucleus still has its expansion power, the annulus already has tears and fissures, and there is a high level of activity, with exposure to external forces in jobs and sports."[7]

Obviously the need for hygienic spinal care is paramount to avoid the inevitable back attack and disc problems. Again, think of spinal exercises as you would of toothpaste as a form of prevention. According to Dr. Pettibone, spinal exercises are important for many reasons:

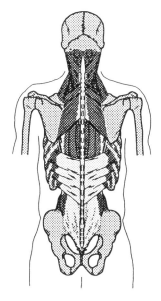

**Superficial
Back Muscles**

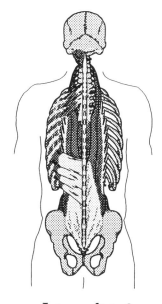

**Intermediate &
Deep Back Muscles**

1. Because they can be used for the control of pain and symptoms.

2. They can be used to establish equal bilateral muscle tonicity, thereby reducing spinal stress and eliminating the "Piezo" electric effect on bone which leads to pathologies like spurs.

3. They are essential in re-establishing and rehabilitating soft tissues that have been damaged through accidents.

4. They are necessary for rehabilitating pathological spinal conditions and paravertebral soft tissues.

5. They can speed recovery and reduce the number of office visits required for the average patient.

6. When done properly, they can continue correction of partially reduced subluxations.

7. They actively involve the patient in his or her own health-care program while doing exercises at home.

Restoration of the spine and the body in general occurs mostly during sleep. It becomes essential to sleep in a posture that allows the entire spine and muscular system to relax, in other words, in order to not support the skeletal system whatsoever. The best sleeping posture is flat on your back with your neck and lumbar spine supported with rolled pillows and with your knees bent in a supported fashion as well. Sleeping on your side causes lateral spinal distortions and does not allow all the muscles to rest. Sleeping on your stomach is a disaster waiting to happen, because your neck is twisted all night, causing the possibility of cervical joint misalignments.

Even after an adjustment, if your spinal muscles are still weak from injury or neglect, putting too much stress on the weakest link in your spine may cause a relapse, as 70 percent of patients discover within six months of their adjustments. To avoid another back attack, you must maintain your spinal stability with periodic adjustments and daily home spinal exercises to improve the muscular strength and joint flexibility of your spine.

For many overweight and deconditioned patients, losing excess body fat also will help immensely. Unfortunately, too many deconditioned, overweight patients don't want to hear that they must change their lifestyles – through exercise and weight reduction – in order to stabilize their weakened backs. They simply want an adjustment to cure them of their back pain forever. Honestly, it just doesn't work that easily. Rehabbing a bad back is no different than rehabbing any joint injury and it takes time and effort to accomplish the best results. I suggest you "get real" about your back attack or else you will definitely suffer another and another and another.

Spinal Threshold Point

Many patients are confused when they come to my office because they don't understand what caused their back to "go out." While a sudden fall, a car accident or other traumatic event explains some causes of back pain, most patients have not experienced these types of traumas in their recent past. After taking care of thousands of cases, I've concluded that most back attacks are accidents just waiting to happen – not unlike Humpty Dumpty sitting on the edge of the wall ready to fall off.

The seeds of patients' back attacks actually were sown years before, when they fell off their bicycles, played football, were thrown off a horse, had a car accident or some other traumatic event in their youth. These accidents went unseen, uncorrected and forgotten, and only worsened as the years went by. Unfortunately, most youthful spinal accidents are never analyzed by a chiropractor, and most children have never had their spines adjusted to correct these seeds for spinal disasters later in life. Spinal misalignments gradually worsen, and combined with a deconditioned state later in life, these minor problems grow into major back attacks when the patient's spinal threshold point is surpassed. Patients wonder why they had a back attack, when in fact, it was a situation similar to the proverbial *"straw that finally broke the camel's back."*

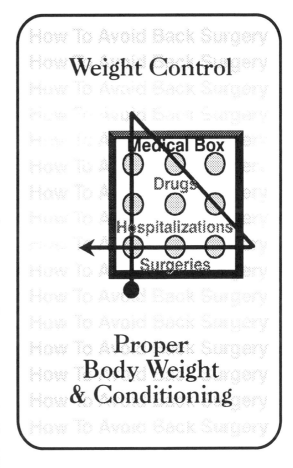

Furthermore, the cause of a low back attack is not always an injury, according to Canadian researchers in a recent study of over 11,000 patients.[8] Actually, this study concluded that as many as 66 percent of patients with low back pain had a spontaneous onset. Researchers stated, "Low back pain is generally not precipitated by a clearly defined injury. Only about one-third of patients who are not involved in Workers' Compensation, insurance claims or pending litigation can identify an event that triggered their back problems. Spontaneous onset is the natural history of most back pain."

If your back has finally "gone out" from years of abuse, neglect, and mistreatment, don't fool yourself into believing it just happened without cause. Think of all the childhood falls, sports injuries, car accidents, and the general strains your back has endured throughout your lifetime. As you gracefully age, the supportive muscles have become weaker and weaker until finally the slightest event can cause the spine to finally "go out." But it was an event that took years to accomplish, and it is an injury that will take time to repair. There are no "quick-fixes" to serious spinal problems.

The key to recovery is to raise the inherent threshold level of your spine. I believe stabilizing a spine is a matter of reaching a threshold point where the spine has enough alignment, strength and flexibility to withstand the stress and forces in your lifestyle. Only when an injured spine has better alignment of the vertebrae and pelvic bones, more strength of the six layers of spinal muscles, and better flexibility and joint play in the 137 joints, can we expect it to become more stable and less painful.

As the patient's spinal alignment, strength and joint flexibility improves, stability and improved function will slowly occur. This threshold point of stability is the turning point in recovery. Compression of the spinal column increases dramatically with excess body weight (some researchers believe every pound of body weight increases the compression of the vertebrae tenfold). Recovery in patients who are overweight, out-of-shape, and generally deconditioned depends upon substantial weight loss before their threshold point is reached. Considering that 75 percent of Americans are overweight and deconditioned, obesity is a major problem in the management of back pain.

Until the threshold point is reached through weight loss, spinal adjustments and spinal exercises, most patients experience relapse due to spinal instability -- one day they feel good, the next day they are in pain again. Until they reach this threshold point and maintain it through daily spinal care, stability will be elusive and relapse is inevitable. A football knee joint will not become stable until it reaches this same threshold point, and this is true for your spinal joints.

Rehabilitating a spine is a very difficult process that requires daily effort; otherwise the spine will not stabilize and may relapse when the slightest "straw" is placed upon it. These so-called spontaneous onsets are actually the "final straws" from years of stresses and strains that your spine has endured. Back attacks don't just happen; they are the result of years of neglect and abuse, not unlike heart attacks.

Daily activities place a certain level of stress on your spine, and if your spinal integrity is normal and you have a high threshold point, your spine can perform well without pain or problems and without an incidence of spontaneous onset back pain. If your spine suffers a force it cannot withstand and exceeds its threshold point, then you will suffer a spinal injury and possible misalignments. In other words, your spinal joints and muscles will not be able to withstand excessive force, such as a fall or whiplash injury, and your spinal column will absorb the force and be damaged, muscles strained and spinal joints sprained, causing a vertebral subluxation. Once this injury happens, your threshold point is lowered and your normal daily activities will become painful. The goal of a spinal rehabilitation program is to raise your threshold point by improving your joint alignment, muscular strength and increasing your normal joint flexibility once again.

Scoliosis

It should be common knowledge that chiropractic care helps with childhood scoliosis,[9-11] but unfortunately, it's not. Not only does chiropractic care help with many childhood problems like asthma,[12-16] colic,[17] enuresis,[18] and otis media,[19-23] but it can help to prevent the commonplace childhood falls and spinal accidents from developing into scoliosis and becoming the seeds for adult problems later. Most spinal problems I have found in adult patients actually began in their youth, when they fell off bicycles, played sports or had one of the multitude of accidents that children normally experience. Unfortunately, these initial spinal mishaps go unseen and uncorrected for years. Then, as adults these patients enter my office, perplexed as to why they are in pain. That's why I am adamant that all children be checked by a professional chiropractor for scoliosis, and not merely by some elementary school teacher who screens her students occasionally. That is equivalent to checking your

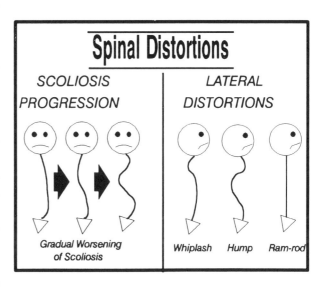

children for dental decay by having a teacher say "smile" to see any problems. Only a professional DC can determine the real extent and severity of scoliosis and do something to help it.

How scoliosis develops is a mystery to many. While a small percentage of patients may have deformed vertebrae at birth, in most cases scoliosis is a slow developmental process that starts with early misalignments. For example, when a child falls, usually the pelvis becomes distorted first. The tailbone (sacrum) generally falls off the level and then acts to cause the lumbar spine to tilt to the left or right. This is called the "leaning tower look," when the head is leaning to one side dramatically off-center. If this goes uncorrected, the next phase is the "C" shape scoliosis, where the head is back centered over the pelvis, but the spine is now curved like the letter "C." This phase is seen a lot in young children or with fresh injuries in adults. If this phase is uncorrected, the spine evolves to the next, more stable phase, which is the double "S" curve, generally seen in young adults who originally damaged their spines in their youth. It takes a few years for this curve to develop, so it is usually seen in mid-life. Lastly, if this phase is uncorrected, the spine will develop into the triple "S" curve, which is normally seen in senior citizens. This evolution of scoliosis is inevitable if the underlying cause is not corrected and properly managed. Just as your teeth need lifetime care from childhood on, so does your spine.

In a side view of your spine, ideally there are four curves – two that bow forward (lordotic) in the neck (cervical) and low back (lumbar) spine, and two that bow backwards (kyphotic) in the mid-back (dorsals) and the tailbone (sacrum). These curves actually make your spinal column stronger as a weight-bearing unit to support the head and torso and resist gravity. But when accidents occur, these normal curves are distorted as well. Typically a rear-end collision will reverse the lordotic curve in the neck and cause it to bend backwards – classic "whiplash." But don't think that only car accidents can cause this reverse curvature. Passive activities like sitting in a chair for hours in front of a computer also slowly distort your natural spinal curves, decondition the spinal muscles and lead to scoliotic problems in children and adults. There are many ways to distort your spine in your youth or as an adult. The important point is that you and your children should be checked by a chiropractor regularly to stop or reverse this process.

And it doesn't get any easier for most kids. Who hasn't fallen out of a crib, off the bed or swingset? What child doesn't fall while learning to skate or bike? And for the more active children, sports can cause a multitude of spinal accidents. Actually, some of the worst cases of whiplash injury I have seen have not only been car accidents, but serious falls from bicycles and horses. And let's not even talk about motorcycles – or as I call them, "murdercycles."

As you can imagine, and as many of you may have experienced, spinal injuries are commonplace on playground and in organized sports. Is it little wonder that estimates say 90 percent of all football players will have lifetime spinal problems, considering the trauma inflicted in every single play? Sports are fun to watch, but they can be tragic to the body, especially the spinal column.

Unfortunately, concern for children's spinal health is largely ignored by parents. As an example of parents mismanaging their children's spinal problems, an unfortunate example came to my office recently. The father, a patient of mine for 15 years himself, brought his teenage son complaining of mid-back pain to my office. Actually, I've watched his son grow up. When the father came to my office for his regular maintenance care, I would suggest that his son get checked as well, but the father would always decline, saying "He's OK, he's not in any pain like me."

In response, I told the father, "That's like waiting until your son has a toothache before you introduce him to toothpaste and dentistry. Why won't you simply let me give him a thorough scoliosis screening to see what's going on in his spine?" The underlying hesitation was more a financial consideration than anything else, because the father and mother were long-time chiropractic patients. Unfortunately, their cost-consciousness lead to bigger problems years later for their son.

When the son was 16 years old, he finally had his inevitable back attack, and upon x-ray examination of his spine, I found this boy had severe "S" shape scoliosis due to a tilted sacrum and a short-leg syndrome. I was stunned to see how severe his spinal distortions actually were in terms of degrees of curvature as well as initial signs of disc degeneration. Obviously by the overall severity, this scoliosis had been developing for some time. I couldn't contain my rage over this situation because I had warned his parents years before, only to be put off by them because they didn't see the need or want to pay the price. At the Report of Findings, I flatly told his father, "This is your fault!" His son's severe scoliosis was due to his parents' neglect to let me check him when he was younger when this condition could have been circumvented with corrective care. Instead, to save a few dollars, they neglected his spinal health only for him to suffer the consequences later.

Let this example be a warning to every parent: Don't neglect your children's spinal health. Just as you have their teeth checked and cared for regularly, please do the same for your children's spines. Afterall, what's more important – their teeth or their spinal column? For your children's sake, I hope you get my point.

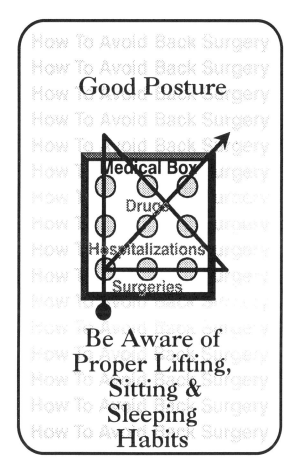

Safe in Skilled Hands

Unfortunately, the medical scare stories and slanderous remarks about chiropractors "cracking" necks have frightened many potential patients from chiropractic care. Some patients tell me they envisioned some type of chiropractic karate or some sort of "Hulk Hogan, DC," who would slam-dunk them on an adjusting table. This fear has kept many people from enjoying the benefits of spinal care and has lead to many unnecessary surgeries as well. When I ask patients if they are scared about their first adjustment, knowing that many are, I ask them why they are nervous. Most often their medical doctor has scared them with slanderous remarks: *"Don't go to a chiropractor or he'll paralyze you."* If you were to believe these medical bigots, you might think everyone is hurt by chiropractors, which is the furthest thing from the actual truth.

Can you imagine the *voo-doo* salesmanship it must take to scare a patient about a simple spinal adjustment, and then to sell them a dangerous and ineffective back surgery? But for the most part, adjustments don't hurt and actually feel great, that's why patients keep coming back. As many tell me, adjustments are "addictive" because they do feel so good. As one patient who is a dentist once said to me, *"You chiropractors have it easy, because your treatment feels so good, unlike mine."*

Although many medical detractors frighten patients about chiropractic adjustments by talking about "cracking," "snapping" or "twisting your neck," implying forceful, harmful treatments, the facts show just the opposite. We chiropractors prefer the term "adjustment" to any other term, including "manipulation," because it signifies something more controlled, specific and skilled. Actually, a chiropractic spinal adjustment is considered technically to be a specific, high-velocity, short-lever, low-amplitude thrust into the joints of the spine. Other manual manipulators, like osteopaths and physical therapists, may render manipulations which usually are very forceful, slow-velocity, long-lever and non-specific. There is a huge difference between a specific adjustment of individual spinal segments and a non-specific manipulation of regional areas of the spine. I've had patients come to me after their local MD or PT has tried to manipulate them, only hurting them with his or her non-specific wrenching of their necks or low backs. It's quite ironic that some MDs will scare patients about the supposed dangers of chiropractic adjustments in the hands of a skilled DC who has practiced this technique for years, and then take it upon themselves to render a crude imitation without any training or experience whatsoever..Go figure!

The question about the nature and safety of a chiropractic adjustment was addressed by the New Zealand Commission's Inquiry on Chiropractic:

"[I]t is alleged that [chiropractic] techniques consists mainly of the 'dynamic thrust'. This is claimed to be dangerous because it is a sudden high-velocity movement, the patient cannot see what is being done, cannot resist the thrust, and is therefore at the chiropractor's mercy.

"... we find it reasonable to suppose that any known cases of harm caused by chiropractic treatment would have been brought to our attention. We learned of only three.

"Until the Commission saw chiropractors at work, it imagined from such descriptions that this was the only way the chiropractor operated, while the physiotherapist, with gentle articulations, extension, or mobilization was a very different practitioner. The truth is that, while the chiropractor's movements are indeed often quick, perhaps more so than those of the physiotherapist, they are also usually small and precise. **The most forceful manipulations we saw were performed by physiotherapists.**"[24]

The Manga Report from Ontario (Canada) Ministry of Health also addressed this issue, inasmuch as it found that adverse reactions to adjustments "have been used as a weapon against chiropractors."

"The safety of chiropractic manipulation has been closely scrutinized, sometimes with evident bias... However the relative safety of chiropractic manipulation is amply documented and studied... Our reading of the literature suggests that chiropractic manipulation is far safer than medical management of LBP.

"The literature review generated a rather curious overall conclusion. While it is prudent to call for even further clinical evidence of the effectiveness and efficacy of chiropractic management of LBP, what the literature revealed to us is the much greater need for clinical evidence of the validity of medical management of LBP. Indeed, several existing medical therapies of LBP are, on the basis of the existing clinical trials, generally contraindicated. **There is also some evidence in the literature to suggest that manipulations are less safe and less effective when performed by non-chiropractic professionals.**"[25]

The recent AHCPR Guideline for Acute Low Back Pain in Adults also mentions the safety issue in the brochure guide for patients which states, "This treatment (using hands to apply force to the back to 'adjust' the spine) can be helpful for some people in the first month of low back symptoms. **It should only be done by a professional with experience in manipulation.**"[26]

Even the esteemed orthopedic author, Dr. Ruth Jackson, writes in her textbook titled, *The Cervical Syndrome*, about the benefits of spinal manipulation, warning that it is best done by experienced practitioners only: "There are many manipulators who manipulate the cervical spine and who claim excellent results...Manipulation of the cervical spine should not be undertaken by any person who is not well versed in the anatomy of this very complex structure. Neck popping has resulted in severe neurological problems, some near fatal and others fatal."[27]

The recurring theme of these investigators is that spinal adjustments are extremely safe and

The Solution to Back Pain

Medical Box

Drugs

Hospitalizations

Surgeries

Spinal Adjustments, Exercises, Weight Loss & Good Posture

effective in the hands of chiropractors. Don't be fooled into believing that they are painful or dangerous. The facts are clear that spinal manipulation is safe in the hands of a skilled professional – a chiropractor. Keep in mind: Any tool works best in skilled hands.

Let me try to clarify this concern about the supposed dangers of manipulation of the neck causing strokes. First of all, a stroke is a dietary problem due to years of junk food accumulation. Secondly, researchers have stated that more people develop strokes from washing their hair over a sink, backing out of their driveway, doing yoga, calisthenics, overhead work, star gazing, archery or bending the neck for a bleeding nose than they would from an adjustment. Actually, you have a much higher chance of being hit by lightning (one in 600,000) than you do having a stroke as a result of an adjustment.

During the medical media misinformation campaign about strokes, many other relevant facts about this issue failed to appear in print despite their importance. For instance, the rate of incidence of stroke from manipulation has been estimated to be one or two cases in 1,000,000 patients, but if you read these newspaper articles or saw biased television reports such as ABC's news program, "20/20," you might have thought that most patients leaving a chiropractic office were suffering from a stroke. Nothing could be further from the truth.

Not only was the minute ratio of problems not mentioned in the news releases, but the media also failed to mention that the medical procedures (neck surgeries) have a rate of 15,000 accidents per million! Even more significant, the researchers proved that 40 percent of these accidents caused by manipulation are caused by non-DC practitioners![28] This means that the 6 percent of manipulations performed by MDs, PTs, and DOs accounted for 40 percent of the problems. But this fact failed to make the news articles and would have been very embarrassing for the medical community. Instead, chiropractors have been made out to be the fall guys and held to blame for accidents caused by others. It never ceases to amaze me how the medical media distorts the truth to mislead people. So, the next time you hear an MD scaring people about chiropractic care, remember the actual truth about who's hurting patients and you'll realize that your MD is deceiving you. And we wonder why we have a health-care crisis, when the truth is so hard to come by!

Even Dr. Philip R. Lee, HHS assistant secretary for health and head of the U.S. Public Health Service, stated, "Our intent is not to scare people away from chiropractic manipulations. Indeed, most interventions by allopathic physicians have a higher complication rate than chiropractic interventions."[29]

Another medical researcher, Jeffrey Jentzen, MD has said, "Based on the approximately 11 million cervical manipulations reported to be performed in this country each year, I would place the incidence of lethal stroke syndrome following cervical manipulation at about one in one million."[30]

The cover-up by the media of the problems with neck and back surgery and its embellishment of the incidence of chiropractic accidents is another example of its biased reporting. If the media wants to discuss iatrogenic problems, why does it limit its discussions to only problems caused by chiropractors and spinal manipulations? Why does it fail to inform the public that 1,600 children will die this year from allergic reactions to aspirin alone? Or that Prozac will kill more than that? Or that 1.5 million people will be hospitalized this year from iatrogenic reactions and over 100,000 die each year in American hospitals due to medical mistakes? Over 1,000 people will die every week from unnecessary surgery, while their doctors explain, *"The operation was a success, but the patient died."* Actually, medical malpractice is now the third leading cause of death in America killing over 150,000 yearly, yet the media has been strangely quiet on this issue.[31]

Obviously, in comparison to most medical methods, chiropractic adjustments are incredibly safe. A good chiropractic spinal adjustment feels great and is safe 99.999 percent of the time. People who have never had their spines adjusted don't know how good they can actually feel. In many cases, immediate pain relief occurs, joint play is restored allowing for better range of motion, pressure on pinched nerves is relieved and an immediate improvement is experienced. While immediate relief does not always occur, especially in acute traumatic cases or in chronic cases of neglect, most patients feel better after an adjustment. As the old chiropractic saying goes: *"When your spine is in line, you'll feel fine."* It is a truism more profound than you may realize.

Sour Grapes, AMA!

With the avalanche of governmental recommendations of spinal manipulation for the epidemic of low back pain, the AMA's response has been less than enthusiastic to say the least. Not only did a group of orthopedic surgeons attempt to block the release of the AHCPR guideline on acute low back pain, their eventual acknowledgement of the recommendations typified their myopia on this matter. In his response to the AHCPR news release, Edward Handley, MD, orthopedic surgeon and spokesman for the Academy of Orthopedic Surgeons, found it quite difficult to congratulate the chiropractic profession. He justified his group's initial decision to withhold endorsement of the new guideline by saying, "My personal view is that the guideline absolutely reflects what science we know, and it is fair and appropriate. But medicine is an art and not just a science. It must not only take into account the scientific literature, but also clinical experience and other factors as well. Just because a particular treatment method [back surgery] has not been proven efficacious does not necessarily mean it is invalid or harmful."[32]

If this isn't sour grapes, I don't know what is. The researchers did take into account every possible reasonable solution to this epidemic of back pain and honestly concluded that manipulation works best in most cases, whereas disc surgery is helpful in only one in 100 cases. Even in light of the changing tide in this area, many surgeons continue to rationalize and mismanage patients through their ineffective methods. Obviously, the truth is hard to come by for the average patient seeking the best possible spinal care. That's one reason why this book was written and it's also the reason why low back pain is considered a 20th century health-care disaster.

After the RAND Corporation and the AHCPR reports on low back pain credited spinal manipulation as being effective, it was ironic – almost unbelievable – to see the medical world attempt to claim expertise in this area. I recall on ABC's "World News Tonight," whose medical reporter, Timothy Johnson, MD, reporting on the RAND study, had the audacity to tell the American public that chiropractors weren't the sole proprietors of spinal manipulation. On NBC's "Today Show," their medical reporter, Art Ulene, MD, also distorted the truth of the AHCPR guideline by recommending the public use DOs instead of DCs. In fact, if the art of spinal manipulation had been left in the hands of DOs, this great healing method would have become a lost art. For the most part, osteopaths have given up spinal manipulation and have become, in essence, typical medical practitioners using drugs and surgery as their foremost methods, not manipulation.

With the announcement of the AHCPR report, Dr. Stanley Bigos, head of the 23-member panel, could not bring himself to endorse chiropractors when he said the same thing – that spinal manipulation was done by medical people as well as by chiropractors. Since the RAND report itself mentions that chiropractors perform 94 percent of all spinal manipulations (osteopaths, physical therapists and medics perform only 6 percent), their statements can only be viewed by chiropractors as disingenuous, to say the least, and downright hypocritical, to tell the honest truth.

Apparently these medical men just cannot give credit where credit is due. When it comes to either specific spinal adjustments or general spinal manipulation, chiropractors are, by far, the masters of this art. A recent survey by the Foundation for Chiropractic Education and Research (FCER) has revealed that chiropractors receive the most training in spinal manipulation when compared to other health-care providers:[33]

Chiropractic students	– 563 hours
Osteopathic students	– 146 hours
Medical students	– 0 hours
Physical therapy students	– 0 hours

In light of the fact that DCs have three times the training as DOs in spinal manipulation and considering the fact that MDs and PTs have no academic training whatsoever in this healing art, the public should be aware of the lack of expertise by anyone other than DCs. After the AHCPR news release, Dr. Lowry Morton, Chairman of the board of governors of the ACA, mentioned the possibility of non-qualified chiropractic imposters:

"While this exciting new study shows spinal manipulation to be effective for the treatment of back problems, I am concerned that these positive findings may lead many non-qualified technicians to jump on the band wagon and try to administer some sort of spinal manipulation. While spinal manipulation is safe in the hands of a doctor of chiropractic, who is trained to perform the procedure, I would not take the risk of putting myself in the custody of a non-skilled individual. With every major success comes those who try to take advantage of a situation – the imitators and imposters."[34]

The latest wrinkle in this confusion are books which offer do-it-yourself courses in manipulation and weekend courses being sold to teach non-qualified individuals manipulative procedures! The outright hypocrisy of the medical world is incredible. After a century of criticizing spinal manipulation as a form of treatment, even in the hands of highly trained chiropractors, and scaring patients with their unfounded *voo-doo* threats, some medical people suddenly feel ready to render this highly-skilled method of spinal adjusting after a weekend seminar. After a century of cheap shots at chiropractic, now that the research verifies the effectiveness of spinal manipulative therapy, they want to jump on our bandwagon.

Gimme a break!

Fortunately, a recent legal decision has taken the first action to protect patients from these pretenders. Kansas Attorney General Carla Stovall has issued a formal opinion stating that "...chiropractic manual manipulation as taught in accredited schools of chiropractic is not within the scope of practice of medicine and surgery as defined by K.S.A. 65-2869." The opinion further states: "The legislature clearly intended the distinctions between healing arts branches not be obliterated. K.S.A. 65-2869(g) prohibits a licensee from invading the field of practice of any branch in which the licensee is not licensed to practice." This opinion will also prohibit MDs from directing PTs to perform chiropractic manual manipulations.[35]

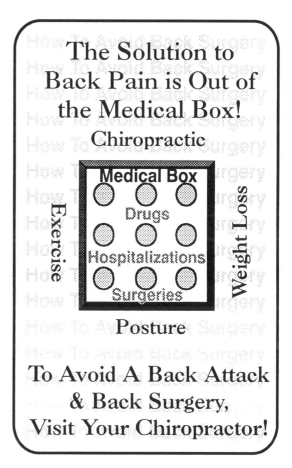

If an MD, PT or DO tries to convince you that he or she can duplicate chiropractic adjustments, I suggest you consult a chiropractor instead. Not only did RAND confirm that chiropractors do the majority of spinal adjustments, it confirmed that DCs do it nearly 100 percent of the time, whereas those few MDs, DOs and PTs who attempt spinal manipulation do it only a fraction of their time. Comparing PTs to DCs is like comparing an optician to an ophthalmologist – while they both deal with the same area of the body, their skills and intentions are quite varied. Would you rather have someone adjusting your spine who does it 100 percent of their time in practice, or someone who does it only occasionally? Would you rather have someone who has studied and practiced this art exclusively or someone who is really untrained and disinterested in spinal adjusting anyway? Who are the real experts and who are the real pretenders? It's obvious that chiropractors are the real experts when it comes to spinal care and the best solution to America's number one health-care problem. Consumer beware!

Not All Chiropractors Are The Same

Once you've made the decision to contact a local chiropractor for care, keep in mind that all DCs are not the same, because there are different types of chiropractic practitioners. Traditional chiropractic adjustors use their hands to adjust the joints of the spine and pelvis. Gonstead, Palmer and Diversified techniques are a few of the larger methods they employ. Other systems of adjusting the spine include Pettibone, Cox, Grostic, Activator or Thompson and use special tables or adjusting instruments to help adjust the joints of the spine. More recently, other methods have emerged which don't physically adjust the joints by hand, but which may use reflex or pressure methods to align the spinal joints. These methods are called B.E.S.T., Nimmo, SOT, DNFT, Logan Basic or Toftness, to name a few.

Other DCs may be skilled at adjusting the joints of the wrists, jaws, ankles, shoulders and knees, to name but a few of the many 300+ joints in the body that can misalign. According to the Occupational Safety and Health Administration (OSHA), repetitive stress injuries (RSI) cost industry over $100 billion annually in lost wages and productivity, and most of these are joint injuries such as back problems, neck, shoulder, elbow and wrist pains due to repetitive usage.[36] OSHA officials admit that every job is a RSI waiting to happen, but medical care hasn't proven effective in treating these cases, since drugs and surgery rarely help mechanical joint problems. If you suffer from RSI problems, I urge you to seek a DC skilled in adjusting the many joints of the skeletal system. If you suffer from jaw pain (TMJ) or wrist pain (carpal tunnel syndrome), seek a chiropractor adept at extremity adjusting before you decide to live on drugs or undergo ineffective surgery. You'll be amazed how simply effective manipulation is for these RSI problems.

One word of caution to the prospective patient: If you do not get good results with one DC, don't think that all DCs are alike. Just as MDs differ in their specialities and skill levels, so are DCs different in their methods and skill levels. Too often a patient may be mis-matched with a DC whose method may not be best suited for that patient's problem. Rather than thinking that all DCs practice the same, I urge you to visit another type of DC who uses a different method. I take care of many transfer patients from other DCs who simply needed a different approach to their problem. And sometimes it does become an issue of skill level when one DC is more skilled at a particular method of adjusting. Just as all baseball players do not possess the same skill level in the game, not all chiropractors are at the same skill level either. So, if you have tried one DC who was unable to help you, don't think to yourself, "I tried chiropractic once and it didn't work." I urge you to try another DC who may be more skillful or who may use a different method or additional rehab equipment.

It may also be a case of cross-purposes between the doctor and patient. If an impatient patient wants a "quick-fix" adjustment, he or she may be disappointed if the doctor operates a comprehensive spinal rehab program and recommends months of care to stabilize a deconditioned spine. These "911" type of patients generally want an immediate cure without any follow-up care or even spinal exercises. Maintenance care is usually out of the question with these prodigal patients who only show up when they have another relapse. In effect, these reactive patients are searching for a "chiropractic emergency room." They are looking for the "wonder" adjustment that will instantly and forever cure their back problems. The truth is it simply doesn't happen that way – rehabilitating a spine is a long process that requires time and effort to stabilize and "quick-fixes" just aren't realistic for spinal rehab, whether it's a spinal adjustment or a back surgery.

It's important to find the right type of chiropractic office to meet your needs. Not all DCs are the same in their approach, methods or treatment plans. Some offer complete spinal rehab, some may offer nutritional advice, while others mainly adjust the spine. Many DCs also utilize adjunctive therapies in addition to their adjusting technique. Some DCs operate spinal rehabilitation facilities which use soft tissue modalities to help the muscles and ligaments heal. Ask your friends about the different chiropractic offices and you'll find the right one for you.

There are DCs whose art of practice also involves nutritional advice such as vitamin therapy, herbal or homeopathic remedies, weight control programs or general wellness programs which include natural methods to restore good health. Again, not all DCs simply adjust the spine to help with back pain. Chiropractic is a more holistic approach to natural good health, and many DCs are quite knowledgeable about other methods of natural healing that have been used for hundreds of years. Don't think that chiropractors are only good for back pain or you will be denying yourself a wonderful source of wellness information. You must seek out these exceptional DCs who practice holistic health care, because not every DC does so.

Keep in mind that the practice of chiropractic is varied and very different from the practices of mainstream medical men or physical therapists. Chiropractic is a separate profession because of its distinctive approach to health and treatment. Often people mistakenly think that chiropractic is similar to physical therapy, forgetting that PTs have nothing to do with the science of neurophysiology and that they know little about the art of spinal manipulation. No other profession adjusts the spinal column to remove this cause of pain and neurogenic disease. Stick with the best spinal adjustors – your local doctor of chiropractic. He or she is the best trained, most skilled and most experienced spinal adjustor in the entire health care world. Indeed, the profession of chiropractic is a "diamond" in the world of health-care, but it rests outside the medical box of drugs and surgery. If you want to avoid back surgery and learn how best to manage your spinal column, the chiropractic profession stands ready to serve you. Isn't it time that you discovered how this simply amazing art and science might help you become a healthier person?

CHAPTER FIVE

Spinal Research

*"On the evidence, particularly the most scientifically valid
clinical studies, spinal manipulation applied by
chiropractors is shown to be more effective
than alternative treatments for low-back pain."*
– Manga Report
Ontario Ministry of Health

The debate about the effectiveness of chiropractic care has persisted for over 100 years, since its inception in 1895. Despite the millions of satisfied patients who swore about the benefits of spinal adjustments, many medical proponents swore at chiropractors instead, choosing to ignore the obvious benefits of chiropractic care. Without funding for proper research, chiropractic only had millions of anecdotal case successes to justify itself, which were quickly dismissed by the critical scientific community. But within the last decade, many research studies from around the world have investigated chiropractic care as well as medical methods in their quest to solve this epidemic of back problems. Considering the magnitude of positive research supporting spinal manipulation, I dare say we can now pronounce this debate concluded and chiropractic care has won.

The medical world may rue the day when the U.S. Congress and the governments of other nations began research on chiropractic and the epidemic of back pain. Perhaps the medical profession was overly confident in its own beliefs about back pain management or incredibly myopic about those theories of the chiropractic profession, but the call for research into this area caused the federal government to set a new guideline in the management of low back pain. Although they had been given the opportunity to discredit chiropractic's science, to the surprise of everyone except chiropractors, the researchers ended up endorsing spinal manipulation as the best initial form of professional treatment. Indeed, today the medical profession wishes it had kept silent, because without its constant criticism and demand for research, the public would still be in the dark about the best method to manage its spinal problems.

This predicament – the lack of scientific proof – was the reason why political medicine for years remarked that chiropractic care was "unscientific." And to this day, despite the plethora of new research, many MDs who fail to understand the science and logic of chiropractic still choose to ignore the research that does exist. Ironically, there seems to exist a double standard, in that medicine utilizes many treatments that are unproven or unscientific, yet its members rarely criticize themselves. For instance, the Office of Technology Assessment mentioned that only 15 - 20 percent of all medical treatments were proven to be effective, yet medical spokesmen remain strangely quiet on this matter. As P. Joseph Lisa states in his book, *The Assault on Medical Freedom*:

"A report by the Congressional Office of Technology Assessment said that the rest of allopathic medicine is basically a hit-and-miss situation, that allopathic medicine's effectiveness lies in emergency medicine (trauma) and neonatal. The rest of it (80 percent to 85 percent), according to the study, is not effective. Yet America is paying out hundreds of billions of dollars for something that is only 15 percent to 20 percent effective!"[1]

In the studies done on back surgeries, you will read for yourself that the results actually prove their ineffectiveness! When Washington state demands that Workers' Compensation patients sign informed consent releases informing them of the 77 percent failure rates for lumbar fusions, it's obvious that back surgeries have a very limited success rate. Yet the scientific proof that these surgeries are not helpful has never slowed down the surgeons. I imagine it's much easier to throw stones at someone else's glass house than to throw them at your own. But with the multitude of new research from around the world proving spinal manipulation as the most effective treatment for most back pain problems, this criticism comes only from the uninformed or those who stand to profit by rendering unnecessary surgery.

Headache & Migraine Successes

Migraine headaches are excruciating. Anyone who has ever suffered from these terrible pains knows how bad it feels when it seems your brain is swelling beyond the size of your skull. The pain and pressure is beyond description, and this crippling condition plagues millions of people every day. It's no fun having migraine headaches, and it's no fun living with someone who has them. I know all too well, because I grew up with a mother who suffered from these severe headaches. For 30 years my mother lived on every medication on the market, all to no avail. When her only son became a chiropractor, she and my father traveled across the country to visit me. During the entire trip she had her migraine despite the patch of medication her pharmacist had given her. My father flatly said, "If you can help her, please do. She's been no fun to be with on this trip!"

My chiropractic analysis showed she had an upper cervical subluxation along with a lot of spinal arthritis. After only a few adjustments, they left to return home. When they arrived, my mother phoned to tell me she didn't have one headache the entire trip back. A few months later, after seeing her local DC, she phoned again and told me, "I didn't realize how much pain I was in until I got out of it. I thought growing old meant you're suppose to live in pain." While I was happy to hear about her improvement, I mentioned to her, "Can you imagine how your life would have been better if you had gone to a chiropractor 30 years ago?" The point of this story is that no one has to live in pain on useless medication – just visit your chiropractor instead of relying on drugs. Unfortunately, too many people use chiropractic care as their last resort because their MDs and druggists aren't telling them about the possibility of spinal care as an answer to their misery.

Researchers have long known of chiropractic's effectiveness with headaches and migraines, yet few patients are informed about this by their MDs. Migraine headaches are one of the most common neurological disorders, with an estimated prevalence of 5 - 25 percent of people suffering daily. Approximately 70 percent of patients with migraine are women. Not only is there an epidemic of low back problems in our country, but the epidemic of headaches and migraines is just as bad, if not worse. Unfortunately, the common treatment of masking pain with medications is not the answer to either of these problems. The real solution is to correct the underlying cause of the headaches, and in many cases that appears to be focused on the upper cervical spine.

Michael Anthony, MD, a senior Australian neurologist, stated in the *Australian Family Physician*, that one factor of migraine is "cervical spondylosis" with neck stiffness and pain. "When this is recognized appropriate treatment can give impressive results... The aim is to relieve pressure on nerve roots and the upper neck, thereby reducing activation of the spinal tract of the trigeminal nerve, which is part of the pain center in the head and neck... Anti-migrainous drugs are generally not effective in this condition."[2]

Research by doctors of chiropractic into this problem of migraine headaches has proven the important role of spinal adjustments to correct this problem. Howard Vernon, DC, showed that stiffness and pain in the upper cervical spine produced increased nerve activity or "facilitation" in that region. This reduces inhibition or dampening of pain in descending nerve pathways, which in turn, react by constricting blood supply to the head. A migraine results with vasodilation of the extra-carotid supply and pain mediated by the ipsilateral trigeminal nerve.[3]

In 1978, another important chiropractic researcher, J.S. Wight, DC, published an account of chiropractic's effectiveness with headaches dating back to 1928 with success rates of 72 percent and 90 percent. Of 87 patients, 34 of whom were found to have what was then called "common migraine" and 53 of whom had "classical migraine," 85 percent of females and 50 percent of males with common migraine obtained a "greatly improved" condition. For classical migraine sufferers, 78 percent of females and 75 percent of males achieved similar improvement. In those subjects not reporting a greatly improved status after treatment, a reduction of severe attacks was noted in 81 percent of females and 46 percent of males in the common migraine group and 43 percent and 34 percent respectively in the classical migraine group. This success rate was maintained two years after treatment ended, and the improvement rate applied equally to common and classical migraine, and for male and female patients as well.[4]

Also in 1978, Drs. Parker, Tupling and Prior reported a randomized clinical trial of manipulation for migraine. Eighty-five subjects with an average age of 41 years and an average duration of complaint of 19 years were randomly allocated to one of three treatment groups: 1.) chiropractic manipulation; 2.) medical manipulation and 3.) control/mobilization performed by physiotherapists. Seventy percent suffered from common migraine and the rest from classical migraine. An average of seven treatments were delivered in the treatment stage, or just under one per week. The frequency of migraines was reduced by 40 percent in the chiropractic group, 34 percent in the mobilization control and 13 percent in the medical group. Only one of the study's hypotheses achieved statistical significance, namely, the severity of headaches was reduced to a greater level in the chiropractic group.[5]

In 1985, Drs. Droz and Crot reported on a retrospective study of 332 patients with "occipital headache." The average number of treatments rendered to these patients was nine adjustments. Eighty percent of this sample had a clinical result rated as "very good" (greater than 90 percent relief), while 10 percent had a good outcome. The remaining 10 percent had only slight to no relief. They noted that the vast majority of successful cases had no more than 10 to 15 treatments, establishing an upper limit on the effective treatment dosage. They also reported no worsening cases and no adverse effects of spinal manipulation.[6]

In 1987, Drs. Turk and Ratkolb studied 100 cases of chronic non-vascular headache and reported that spinal manipulation to the cervical joints produced clinically significant reduction of headache activity in 75 percent of subjects. Of great interest is the fact that these authors conducted a six-month follow-up and 65 percent of subjects still had significant improvement.[7]

In 1989, Drs. Stodolny and Chmielewski reported on 31 subjects with "cervical migraine." Twenty-four females and seven males with an average age of 48 years were included. The treatment protocol consisted of two to three manual therapy sessions emphasizing manipulation to the cervical spine. After one week, they reported complete relief of headache in 75 percent of subjects. Other findings included a statistically significant increase in range of cervical motion, greatly reduced levels of intersegmental dysfunctions which had been found in 100 percent of subjects at C0-C1 and in 75 percent of subjects at C7-T1, and reductions in dizziness levels in most subjects.[8]

In 1992, Drs. P.D. Boline and C. Nelson reported on a randomized comparative trial of chiropractic manipulation versus the medication amitryptiline in the treatment of tension-type headache. This trial included 150 subjects with an average headache duration of six years. After the six-week/12-treatment intervention stage, subjects in both groups demonstrated clinically and statistically significant reductions of headache activity. However, at the end of a further six-week/no treatment follow-up phase, subjects treated with chiropractic manipulation had significantly less headache activity than those in the drug therapy group.[9]

Overall, the results of these many studies on migraine headaches indicate a high rate of 75 - 90 percent success in the reduction of headache activity after spinal manipulation. Yet, for many headaches sufferers, these findings are rarely ever mentioned to them by their medical physician. Too many people suffer needlessly because their MDs are too quick to prescribe ineffective pain pills, and when that treatment fails, to discount the patients' headaches as "stress" or to tell them, "it's all in your head." Actually, while the pain may be in your head, the source of your headaches starts in your neck. Peter Rothbart, MD, a Toronto anesthetist and pain specialist, admits in regard to headache management that MDs "haven't been much more advanced than Greek physicians were 2000 years ago;" that many headaches thought to be tension headache or migraine are "rooted in neck problems;" and, most candidly, Dr. Rothbart states that "chiropractors were right – many headaches are caused by damaged structures in the neck and scientific evidence proves it."[10]

Whiplash Neck Injury

Another important research study was released in May 1995 by a Quebec Task Force on Whiplash-Associated Disorders entitled, "Redefining Whiplash and its Management." This task force came to similar conclusions as had the U.S. and U.K. inquiries into low back pain management: For neck pain and whiplash disorders, prolonged rest promotes disabilities; passive modalities, muscle relaxants and injection techniques have no proven benefit and NSAIDs or analgesics may be used on a supplementary basis for pain relief. With respect to manipulation, again this task force constantly emphasized that this type of treatment should be done only by appropriately qualified professionals (i.e., chiropractors).[11]

"Neck pain is to the automobile what low-back pain is to the workplace," was the conclusion of these investigators. When you understand the size and weight of the head (like a bowling ball) sitting atop a pillar of small vertebrae (like children's toy building blocks) supported by six layers of ligaments and muscles (similar to rubber bands), when a sudden 2 - 2.5 G's of force is thrust upon this in a split second by a car accident, you can imagine the damage that must occur to the neck. Whiplash is a nasty injury that requires reconstruction of the vertebral joint play as well as re-strengthening of the soft tissues. The best form of treatment is realignment of the vertebral joints by chiropractic adjustments and rehabilitation of the spinal muscles with specific spinal exercises. Together, these two approaches will re-create spinal stability and function.

Unfortunately, the typical medical mismanagement of whiplash – giving pain pills and muscle relaxants to these serious spinal injuries – is as laughable as giving them to a football player who has sustained a serious knee injury. This mismanagement of an acute whiplash spinal injury has lead to chronic disability and escalating costs. The task force found that nearly half (46 percent) of the total cost of whiplash cases comes from the 12.5 percent of patients whose conditions developed into a chronic problem where symptoms persisted beyond six months. Without joint rehabilitation from chiropractic adjustments, no neck will ever be completely healed, leading to a lifetime problem that never gets better. Obviously, every whiplash victim – whether the whiplash is caused by a car accident, bicycle fall or any traumatic injury – should first be treated by a qualified chiropractor who specializes in these complex injuries.

Kids Need Chiropractic Too

Let me state emphatically every child needs regular spinal care, just like they need regular dental care. Spinal care in children is even more essential than dental care, and the sooner it starts the better. The moment a child is born, trauma may occur to its spine. Forceps delivery and the pulling and twisting of the birthing process is enough force to misalign any child's neck. My own children were checked within minutes of their births to correct any initial vertebral subluxations. Unfortunately, most children are not checked and the process of spinal misalignments and nerve interference begins. Only a chiropractor who specializes in child care can properly detect and correct these initial spinal problems. Every child should be checked at birth and regularly thereafter to prevent a spinal malady.

Just think of the birth process itself. In normal cases the baby emits vaginally face down, whereupon the doctor turns the head about 120 degrees to move the shoulders into place to extract the baby. That's quite a twist, and it causes problems when the doctor pulls the baby out. For many infants it's not unlike getting a whiplash at birth. Indeed, spinal misalignments for many people occur at the moment of their birth. In fact, research in 1979 from Harvard Medical School by Dr. Floyd Gilles found a strong correlation between sudden infant death and forceps delivery: Seven out of eight crib deaths were forceps delivery at birth.[12] The extreme extension of the infantile neck, along with the twisting rotational movement is enough to cause severe damage to the brain stem region of the upper cervical spine.

Abraham Towbin, MD and author of another article about the dangers of forceps, titled "Latent Spinal Cord and Brain Stem Injury in Newborn Infants," mentioned some shocking facts about traumatic delivery:

> "The birth process, even under optimal controlled conditions, is potentially a traumatic crippling event for the fetus...the Apgar test, now widely applied after delivery in appraising respiratory action, cardiac function, muscle tone, reflex irritability and other elementary signs in the newborn, is in essence an appraisal of the presence or absence of injury to the brain stem and spinal cord... Yet, paradoxically, the importance of injury at birth to the brain stem and spinal cord are matters which have generally escaped lasting attention.
> "Forceful longitudinal traction during delivery, particularly when combined with flexion and torsion of the vertebral axis, is thought to be the most important cause of neonatal spinal injury... When excessive traction is applied to the fetal spinal column, fracture, dislocation, and cord transaction occurs... Such injury may occur with breech delivery, in applying traction to the trunk and in manipulating the aftercoming head, or in cephalic delivery when forceps traction is applied. Two mechanisms of trauma are involved: stretch-injury and pressure-injury. With traction there occurs stretching and tearing of surface vessels, of meninges and nerve roots, and tearing and hemorrhage deep within the cord and brain stem... Other forms of mechanical injury occurring during delivery bring about cord compression; vertebral subluxation may occur, often escaping detection.
> "The effect of obstetrical traction was studied experimentally by Duncan (1874), who tested the tensile strength of the spinal column in the fresh term

fetus. He found that in some instances with traction of 90 pounds the vertebral column yielded; the disseverance of the vertebrae invariably took place in the cervical region. Decapitation occurred with 120 pounds of force. Duncan commented 'This is probably far from being what most obstetricians would regard as a great force.'

"The effects of the superimposed cerebral damage may prove far more crippling than that of the primary cord injury; infants so blighted may ultimately manifest symptoms of cerebral palsy, mental retardation, epilepsy or other nervous system disorders.

"It should be noted that between one and two percent, or more, of pregnancies terminate in neonatal death – over 50,000 per year in the United States; findings in the past and in the present material indicate that greater than 10 percent to 33 percent of neonatal cases at autopsy show evidence of spinal or brain stem injury."[13]

Given these facts, any baby born using traumatic methods should be checked immediately for this initial vertebral subluxation by a competent chiropractor. Can you imagine how many babies could have been saved if forceps were not used and if chiropractors immediately checked them? Unfortunately, we will never know.

Actually, new research has indicated that the use of alternative medicine by children is increasing. An article titled, "The Use of Alternative Medicine," by L. Spigelblatt, MD in the *Journal of Pediatrics* reported that "alternative medicine is an aspect of child health that no longer can be ignored." A study determined that 11 percent of those surveyed had taken their children to non-MD providers, mainly chiropractors. The findings also indicated that mothers who chose alternative care were better educated than those who chose conventional medical care. The main reasons for seeking alternative care were for respiratory (27 percent), ENT (24 percent), musculoskeletal (15 percent), skin (6 percent) and prevention (5 percent). The factors influencing choice of using alternative care were word of mouth (23 percent), chronic medical problems (19 percent), dissatisfaction with conventional medicine (14 percent) and more personalized attention (9 percent).[14]

It's well known that children have their common colds, fevers and flus, but few parents realize that many children suffer from spinal pain as well. Modern research has discovered that back pain among children is not only commonplace, it actually plants the seeds for scoliosis and adult spinal problems. A large study of adolescent low back pain in Pennsylvania, published in the *American Journal of Public Health,* confirmed the findings of similar studies performed in Canada, England, and Switzerland. The study involved 1,242 adolescent children aged 11 to 17 from an urban school district in Pennsylvania. It concluded that 30.4 percent reported a history of lower back pain, 22 percent with recent pain. One-third of these cases had limitations in activities, and one in four sought treatment. There was a markedly accelerating incidence of low back pain throughout adolescence, and there was an equal incidence of low back pain in boys (30.7 percent) and girls

(30.0 percent).[15]

Other studies in England, Canada and Europe also found sacroiliac dysfunction to be a common cause of low back pain in children. In fact, the frequency of sacroiliac pain was 29.9 percent in elementary pupils, 41.5 percent in secondary school pupils, and one in three children overall suffered from low back pain.[16] Obviously spinal injuries are not reserved for adults only. Most adult problems actually stem from these early spinal mishaps which go misdiagnosed, untreated, or just ignored when the pain subsides. Unfortunately, most parents overlook these childhood spinal injuries, or at best, bring their kids into a chiropractic office years after these accidents occurred. Again, that's equivalent to teaching your children about toothpaste only after they had a toothache – a bit too late!

Actually, spinal decay is more prevalent in children than most people realize. In 1991 a study on low back pain and disc degeneration in children concluded "that disc degeneration is a frequent finding among children with low back pain at the age of 15 years. Asymptomatic disc degeneration also is frequently found in children of this age."[17] A follow-up study by the same researchers in 1995 revealed: "The frequency of disc degeneration at follow-up was greater in the patients with LBP (increased from 42% to 58%) than among the asymptomatic subjects (from 19% to 26%)." They also found disc protrusions evident on MRI exams in patients with LBP increased from 6% to 26%, and patients without pain also increased from 0% to 16%. The researchers concluded that "degenerative changes emerge rapidly after the adolescent growth spurt. The MR imaging appearance of the degenerative processes is similar regardless of symptoms, although these processes are more common in symptomatic adolescents and develop at an earlier age. There appears to be a positive correlation between degenerative lumbar disc disease and LBP in adolescence."[18]

Unfortunately, most Americans haven't bought the idea of giving their spines preventative care. As I said before, this neglect is like never brushing your teeth or visiting a dentist. Can you imagine what bad shape your teeth would be in by now? Of course, patients cringe at the thought of not giving their teeth daily maintenance care, but they just have never learned to give their spines the same consideration. I believe this negligence is primarily due to the fact that people cannot see spinal distortions and decay as they can see dental problems and decay. In other words, spinal neglect may simply be a matter of "out of sight, out of mind."

Furthermore, uncorrected childhood spinal injuries not only cause immediate problems, but later in life they evolve into serious scoliosis and adult spinal degeneration and weaknesses. Don't neglect having your children checked regularly for spinal problems just as you do for dental problems. As the researchers have proven, disc degeneration is highly prevalent in teenagers, plus the seeds of scoliosis begin in these early days of life.

Don't let this happen to your children. Don't procrastinate to have your children checked by a DC, just as you have a dentist check them regularly for dental problems. And don't rely on MDs or school teachers to detect spinal distortions in your children with superficial visual examinations. Only a professional chiropractor is qualified to give you the best analysis of your family's spinal health. Kids need chiropractic, too!

Low Back Problems

Within the last decade, most spinal research has dealt with the epidemic of acute low back pain in adults because of the overwhelming costs. Since low back problems are the leading cause of disability for people under the age of 45 and are the leading workplace injury, much interest has been given to this costly epidemic. As Dr. Gordon Waddell said, "Low back pain is a 20th century health-care disaster."

The facts associated with back pain are staggering. Statistically, a majority of Americans will suffer some type of spinal injury is a foregone conclusion – the average automobile driver will suffer a serious whiplash spinal injury every 10 years; over 80 percent of all adults will experience a low back attack in their lifetime; a prevalence rate of 30 - 40 percent of Americans suffering with back pain in any given month; a yearly prevalence of symptoms in 50 percent of working-age adults; which amounts to over 34 million cases a year.

The facts also tell us it's getting worse, not better. One estimate of the costs from low back pain alone in the U.S. is in excess of $100 billion per annum. Other U.S. data reveals that 49 percent of time-loss incidents, 67 percent of total time-loss days and an average of 10.8 days lost per incident result from back pain. In addition, back pain has been found to account for the most hospitalizations and surgery in the U.S., with 50 percent of back pain sufferers being hospitalized, 22 percent undergoing surgery for their affliction, and 12 - 14 percent having repeat surgeries. Back problems comprise the third most common Diagnostic Related Group for all hospital discharges, following only natural childbirth and tubal ligations, and back pain is the second most common cause of physical disability after cardiovascular disease. Moreover, it is increasing faster than any other form of chronic disability. Dr. Waddell warns, "We are facing an epidemic of lower back disability in all western societies."

Perhaps most importantly, back injuries have been found to be three times more costly than non-back injuries, and back injury claimants tended to have multiple claims compared to their non-back injury counterparts. Workers' Compensation costs in 1990 alone in the U.S. were estimated at about $30 billion. With the increasing costs associated with these spinal injuries, as well as the poor clinical responsiveness from the traditional medical management, many researchers have investigated this growing concern and have come to conclusions that may surprise people unaware of the new studies.

In 1992 an investigation was conducted by the RAND Corporation and funded by the Foundation for Chiropractic Research and Education. This multi-disciplinary panel of experts conducted a two-year literature review and published its report titled, "The Effectiveness of Spinal Manipulation for Low Back Pain," which basically proved what chiropractors have always known – that spinal manipulation is very effective in the management of low back pain. The RAND study was the first of many reports that sent shock waves through the medical community. The press reported that spinal manipulation is safe, effective and cost-efficient for treatment of low back pain.

For the first time, chiropractic had the stamp of approval from a legitimate research organization. The RAND study also casts doubt on medical methods such as surgery, and it ended the medical criticism that chiropractic was unsubstantiated by research. Paul Shekelle, MD, director of the RAND study, stated:

> "To say that there is no scientific proof, I would say that there's considerably more randomized controlled trials which show benefit for this (spinal manipulation) than there is for many other things which physicians and neurosurgeons do all the time. [19]

> "The data are sufficient to say that spinal manipulation is definitely better than many medical therapies that people used in the past."[20]

Actually, the case for chiropractic care is made quite easy in light of the plethora of new research which has shown chiropractic care to be both clinically superior as well as more cost-effective in the vast majority of non-pathological back problems. You will find quite interesting the numerous exhibits of proof of the superiority of chiropractic care, as well as exhibits of proof against medical methods and back surgery. This sampling is just a handful of the 4,000 articles that convinced the investigators at RAND, Manga and the AHCPR of the benefits of spinal manipulation and chiropractic care.

🄴🅇🄷🄸🄱🄸🅃🅂 🄾🄵 🄿🅁🄾🄾🄵

The Case for Chiropractic Care

🄴🅇🄷🄸🄱🄸🅃 🄸
Department of Health and Human Services
U.S. Public Health Service
Agency for Health Care Policy and Research
Associated Press article

On December 8, 1994, Philip R. Lee, MD, H.H.S. secretary for health and director of the Public Health Service announced new federal guidelines for acute low back pain: "Up to 80 percent of Americans will have a low back problem of some type at least once by age 50, and the condition is the most frequent cause of temporary disability for persons under 45." Dr. Lee also said that low back problems are second only to the common cold as the reason for visiting family or other primary care doctors.

The guidelines suggest that spinal manipulation can be helpful in relieving pain, especially within the first four weeks – and that surgery may be appropriate when there is a serious spinal condition or when people have severe, disabling and persistent sciatica. The guidelines say that overall, surgery benefits only about one in 100 people with acute low back problems.

The 23-member panel found no sound scientific basis for certain treatment methods, including spinal traction, TENS, acupuncture, lumbar corsets, support belts and back machines.

The panel also did not find evidence of effectiveness to justify potential risks of harmful side effects for extended bed rest (more than four days), oral steroids, colchicine, antidepressants and phenylbutazones, therapies involving the injection of local anesthetics, corticosteroids or other substances into the back.

The guidelines do not recommend other treatments because the lack of proven benefits cannot justify their costs. These treatments are: heat/diathermy, massage, ultrasound, cutaneous laser treatment and electrical stimulation.

The panel conducted an exhaustive review of over 3,900 studies and held a public meeting in developing the guidelines, which were then reviewed by more than 100 other back care experts and tested in health maintenance organizations, private and group practices and occupational medicine clinics.

The panel consisted of experts in orthopedic surgery, family practice, internal medicine, emergency medicine, physical and rehabilitation medicine, industrial medicine, occupational medicine, neurosurgery, neurology, neuroradiology, rheumatology, osteopathic medicine, orthopedic research, community health nursing, chiropractic, physical therapy and occupational therapy, and a consumer representative with acute low back problem experience.

🄴🅇🄷🄸🄱🄸🅃 🄸🄸
The RAND Corporation Study

RAND, the world renowned "think tank," in conjunction with the UCLA Department of Medicine, completed a multidisciplinary study in 1991 and found that spinal manipulation is appropriate for the majority of acute low back pain. This two-year RAND study concluded that chiropractic management is safe, effective, and surprisingly well documented in numerous research articles. Paul Shekelle, MD, director of the RAND study, mentioned: "To say that there is no scientific proof, I would say that there's considerably more randomized controlled trials which show benefit for this (chiropractic care) than there is for many other things which physicians and neurosurgeons do all the time."

Shekelle, Paul G., et al., RAND Corporation Report, "The Appropriateness of Spinal Manipulation for Low-Back Pain", Santa Monica, Calif. 1992.

🄴🅇🄷🄸🄱🄸🅃 🄸🄸🄸
The British Research Council Report

In 1990, the British government completed a major 10-year study and found that chiropractic care in some areas of health care is clearly superior by as much as a 2 to 1 ratio over anything that medicine has to offer. T.W. Mead, MD, concluded that:

"Our trial showed that chiropractic is a very effective treatment, more effective than conventional hospital out-patient treatment for low-back pain, particularly in patients who had back pain in the past and who had severe problems... The improvements in the patients who were treated by chiropractors was between three quarters and twice as great as it was for patients who had been treated in hospitals... and one of the unexpected findings was that the treatment difference – the benefit of chiropractic over hospital treatment – actually persists for the whole of the three year period... The improvement in back pain was 29 percent greater in the patients treated with chiropractic than in those treated in the hospital outpatient department... It looks as though the treatment that the chiropractors give does something that results in a very long-term benefit.

"Chiropractic treatment was more effective...mainly for patients with chronic or severe pain...with a potential savings of $42 million."

Meade T.W., Dyer S., et al. "Low Back Pain of Mechanical Origin: Randomized Comparison of Chiropractic and Hospital Outpatient Treatment", *British Medical Journal*, 2 June 1990, Vol 300 #67137, pp. 1431-1437.

EXHIBIT IV
HMO Study

The largest HMO in the entire southeastern United States sent 100 of its medically unresponsive patients to a local chiropractor and recorded the results. The HMO found that 86 percent of this group were helped. More importantly, 12 cases out of 12 previously medically diagnosed as needing disc surgery were all corrected within two to three weeks, saving the HMO over $250,000 (notwithstanding the pain, suffering, disability costs and possible future surgeries since 40 percent of these patients require a second back surgery.) Despite these astounding results, many HMOs continue to exclude chiropractic care from their covered treatments.

Silverman M, "Study of the First 100 Patients Referred to the Silverman Chiropractic Center by AV-MED," *The Chiropractic Report*, vol. 2, no. 2, Jan. 1988.

EXHIBIT V
Utah Workers' Compensation Records

Two studies in Utah by Jarvis (1989) and Phillips and Morris (1991) involving over 3,000 Workers' Compensation cases revealed that the cost in lost work days was 10 times less with chiropractic care, and that chiropractic treatment was seven times less costly than medical care. Chiropractic claimants had a higher frequency of return to work within one week or less (40 percent) than medical claimants (29 percent). For the claimants with a history of chronic low back problems, the median time-loss days for MD cases was 34.5 days, compared to nine days for DC cases. The cost difference was just as staggering – medical management of a lumbosacral disc problem cost $8,175 compared to $1,065 for chiropractors managing identical cases.

Jarvis, KB, Phillips, RB, Morris, EK. "Cost per case comparison of back injury claims of chiropractic versus medical management for conditions with identical diagnostic codes." *Journal of Occupational Medicine,* vol. 33, no. 8, pp. 847-852, 1991.

EXHIBIT VI
Wilk vs. AMA
Federal Court Testimony

Per Freitag, MD, an orthopedic surgeon on staff at two Chicago hospitals, only one of which utilized chiropractic care, testified in the Sixth Circuit Federal Court in Chicago during the *Wilk vs. AMA* antitrust trial that the hospital using chiropractic care released patients in half the time of the medical only hospital - - an average of eight days less hospital time and expense. At an average of $650 per day, that's a savings of over $5,000 per patient.

Wilk et al. vs. AMA et al., U.S. Dist. Court (North. Dist. of Ill. East. Div.) No. 76C3777, Getzendanner J, Judgement dated August 27, 1987.

🄴🅇🄷🄸🄱🄸🅃 🅅🄸🄸
University of Saskatchewan Study

World-renowned medical orthopedist Dr. W.H. Kirkaldy-Willis joined forces with chiropractor Dr. David Cassidy in a 1985 research study titled, "Spinal Manipulation in the Treatment of Low Back Pain." Two hundred eighty-eight "totally disabled" patients who had been non-responsive to previous medical care were given two or three weeks of daily spinal manipulation. The results showed the following: 1.) "No restrictions for work or other activities" in 79 percent of 54 patients with posterior facet joint syndrome; 2.) in 93 percent of 69 patients with sacroiliac joint syndrome; 3.) in 88 percent of 48 patients with both syndromes; 4.) in the remaining groups, 36-50 percent of the 112 patients with more serious disorders; and 5.) of 171 patients who had been chronic/disabled for an average of seven years and who were placed under chiropractic care, 87 percent returned to work within three weeks.

Kirkaldy-Willis, WH, Cassidy, JD. "Spinal manipulation in the treatment of low back pain." *Can Fam Physician*, vol. 31, pp. 535-540, 1985.

🄴🅇🄷🄸🄱🄸🅃 🅅🄸🄸🄸
Italian Government Study

The Italian government in 1988 completed a two-year study on over 17,000 patients treated by chiropractors within 22 medical clinics. The university conducting the study found that hospitalization was reduced by 87 percent and work loss by 75 percent through chiropractic care. Imagine the cost savings if every patient had equal access to chiropractic care in America's hospitals.

Postacchini, F., Facchini, M., Pelieri, P. "Efficacy of various forms of conservative treatment in low back pain. A comparative study." *Neuro-Orthop*, vol. 6, pp. 28-35, 1988.

🄴🅇🄷🄸🄱🄸🅃 🄸🅇
Manga Report

Dr. Pran Manga, health economist, was commissioned by the Ministry of Health in Ontario, Canada to review all the international evidence on the management of low back pain. His results shocked the medical community when he concluded:

> "There would be highly significant cost savings if more management of low back pain was transferred from physicians to chiropractors... Many medical therapies are of questionable validity or are clearly inadequate... Chiropractic management is greatly superior to medical management in terms of scientific validity, safety, cost-effectiveness, and patient satisfaction."

Manga, Pran, PhD, et al., "The Effectiveness and Cost-Effectiveness of Chiropractic Management of Low-Back Pain." Ontario Ministry of Health, 1993.

EXHIBIT X
World Congress on Low Back Pain

Dr. J.L. Shaw, orthopedic surgeon, in his speech on low back pain before this interdisciplinary Congress presented his research on 1,000 patients with low back and leg pain which concluded that:

> "98 percent of the patients had a mechanical dysfunction of the sacroiliac joints as the major cause of their low back pain...only two patients required disc surgery.

> "The conventional wisdom is that herniated discs are responsible for low back pain, and that sacroiliac joints do not move significantly and do not cause low back pain or dysfunction. The ironic reality may well be that sacroiliac joint dysfunctions are the major cause of low back dysfunction, as well as the primary factor causing disc space degeneration, and ultimate herniation of disc material.

> "Treatment of these patients by restoration of full sacroiliac joint motion, along with correction of other dysfunctions, led to relief of symptoms in almost all cases. Most remarkable was the absence of need for surgery in these patients."

Shaw, JL, MD, "The Role of the Sacroiliac Joints as a Cause of Low Back Pain and Dysfunction," speech before World Congress on Low Back Pain, University of California, San Diego, Nov. 5-6, 1992.

EXHIBIT XI
"Health Economics and Chiropractic"

This article by Dr. John Dillon, a prominent Australian economist, examines modern health-care economics and concludes:

> "Undoubtedly, in terms of economic appraisal of the current health scene chiropractic is in a very strong position. Compared to medical services, it is an extremely cheap avenue of health-care for those who seek it. Unlike primary medical practice, it does not spiral costs into the system though ancillary and specialist services, hospitalization, and pharmaceuticals. On average, a dollar spent on a chiropractor's services causes no further costs."

Dillon, JL, "Health Economics and Chiropractic," *Annals of the Swiss Chiropractic Association*, vol. VII, pp. 7-17, 1981.

EXHIBIT XII
Florida's Worker's Compensation Study

Dr. S. Wolk, PhD, in a review of 10,000 cases from 1985 to 1987 showed that: 1.) disability was 48.7 percent shorter under chiropractic care; 2.) fifty-one percent of medical patients were hospitalized compared to only 20.3 percent for chiropractic patients; and 3.) the estimated average total cost of care was 83.8 percent higher for the medical group than those under chiropractic care. Treatment costs for patients of chiropractors were significantly lower, at $1,204 per patient compared to $2,213 for patients of physicians.

108

Dr. Wolk concluded that: "The greater number of services provided by chiropractors may ultimately result in less overall cost to the health-care system by reducing the frequency of disabling back injuries and the necessity for more expensive hospital treatment."

> Wolk, S., "Chiropractic vs. medical care: A cost analysis of disability and treatment for back-related workers' compensation cases." *Foundation for Chiropractic Education and Research*, Arlington, VA. Sept. 1988.

🄴🅇🄷🄸🄱🄸🅃 🅇🄸🄸🄸
Manipulation of Patients with Laminectomy

In the RAND research, two case series reported success of chronic low back pain in patients with previous laminectomies. In the series by Potter (1977), prior laminectomy did not alter the response of patients to manipulation with chronic low back pain, with or without neurological findings. Drs. Kirkaldy-Wills and Cassidy (1988), reported a 72 percent response rate in patients without prior laminectomy and a 64 percent response rate in patients with prior laminectomy for patients with chronic back pains of all kinds.

> Potter, GE, "A Study of 744 Cases of Neck and Back Pain Treated with Spinal Manipulation," *Journal of the Canadian Chiropractic Association*, 1977, pp. 154-156.
> Kirkaldy-Willis, WH and JD Cassidy, "Spinal Manipulation in the Treatment of Low-Back Pain," *Canadian Family Physician*, vol. 31, 1975, pp. 535-540.

🄴🅇🄷🄸🄱🄸🅃 🅇🄸🅅
Reduction of Disc Prolapse by Manipulation

Mathews and Yates (1969) studied the effect of manipulation on the reduction of lumbar disc prolapses. Results of this study suggested that small disc protrusions were diminished in size when patients had manipulation as a treatment. The authors concluded that "treatment by manipulation relieved the symptoms of lumbago and repeat epidurography showed that the prolapses were reduced in size."

> Mathews, JA and DAH Yates, "Reduction of lumbar disc prolapse by manipulation," *British Medical Journal*, vol. 3, p. 696, 1969.

🄴🅇🄷🄸🄱🄸🅃 🅇🅅
Treatment of Lumbar Disc Protrusions by Manipulation

An article titled, "Treatment of lumbar intervertebral disc protrusion by manipulation," (1987) by Pang-Fu Kuo and Z. Loh indicated that spinal manipulation was impressive in disc cases. From 1975 through 1983, a total of 517 patients with protruded lumbar discs were admitted for manipulative treatment. Of these, 76.8 percent had satisfactory results. There were 73 recurrences (14.1 percent) at intervals ranging from two months to 12 years. Forty-seven cases did not respond to manipulation. These results indicate that manipulation of the spine can be effective treatment for lumbar disc protrusions.

Kuo, PP, and ZC Loh, "Treatment of lumbar intervertebral disc protrusion by manipulation," Clinical Orthopaedics and Related Research, vol. 215, pp. 47-55, 1987.

🄴🅇🄷🄸🄱🄸🅃 🅇🅅🄸
Manipulation for Disc Herniation

An 1989 article in the *Journal of Manipulative and Physical Therapeutics*, by J. Quon and Dr. J. Cassidy, described the case of a patient with lumbar disc herniation who underwent a course of side posture manipulation. Despite the appearance of an enormous central herniation on the CT scan, the patient improved considerably during only two weeks of treatment. It is emphasized that manipulation has been shown to be an effective treatment for some patients with lumbar disc herniation. While complications of this form of treatment have been reported in the literature, such incidents are rare.

Quon, JA, Cassidy, JD, et al., "Lumbar intervertebral disc herniation: treatment by rotational manipulation." *Journal of Manipulative and Physiological therapeutics*, vol. 12, no. 3, pp. 220-227.

🄴🅇🄷🄸🄱🄸🅃 🅇🅅🄸🄸
Mandated Health Insurance Coverage for Chiropractic Treatment: An Economic Assessment with Implications for the Commonwealth of Virginia.

Executive Summary:

1.) Mandated chiropractic coverage has minimal cost-increasing effects on insurance and may even reduce costs.

2.) The low-cost impact of chiropractic is due not to its low rate of use, but to its offsetting impact on costs in the face of high rates of utilization. Chiropractic is a growing component of the health-care sector, and it is widely used by the population.

3.) Formal studies on the cost, effectiveness or both of chiropractic, usually measured against other forms of treatment, show a favorable comparison.

4.) By every test of cost and effectiveness, the general weight of evidence shows chiropractic to provide important therapeutic benefits at economical costs. Additionally, these benefits are achieved with apparently minimal, even negligible impacts on the costs of health insurance.

5.) The conclusion of this analysis is that chiropractic insurance mandates help make available health care that is widely used by the American public and has proven to be cost-effective.

Schifrin L.G. "Mandated Health Insurance Coverage for Chiropractic Treatment: An Economic Assessment with Implications for the Commonwealth of Virginia." The College of William and Mary, Williamsburg, Va., and the Medical College of Virginia, Richmond, Va., Jan 1992.

EXHIBIT XVIII
California Worker's Retrospective Study

In 1975, a 1972 retrospective study of 629 Workers' Compensation cases in California by Dr. C. Richard Wolf was published. It showed that doctors of chiropractic are twice as effective as medical physicians in treating comparable injuries and in returning injured workers to work at every level of injury severity: 1.) average lost time per employee – 32 days in the MD-treated group, 15.6 days in the chiropractor-treated group; 2.) employee reporting no lost time – 21 percent in the MD-treated group, 47.9 percent in the chiropractor-treated group; 3.) employees reporting lost time in excess of 60 days – 13.2 percent in the MD-treated group, 6.7 percent in the chiropractor-treated group.

Wolf, C.R., MD, "Industrial Back Injury," *International Review of Chiropractic,* 26:6-7, Jan. 1974.

EXHIBIT XIX
Oregon Workmen's Compensation Retrospective Study

In 1972, Roland A. Martin, MD, medical director of the Oregon Workmen's Compensation Board, published a study, again based on a retrospective study of comparable workmen's industrial injures, and independently concluded that same 2 to 1 advantage of chiropractic care.

Examining the forms of conservative therapy which the majority received, it is interesting to note the results of those treated by chiropractic physicians. A total of 29 claimants were treated by no physician other than a chiropractor. Of these workers, 82 percent resumed work after one week of time-loss. Their claims were closed without a disability award.

Of the examining claims treated by the MD, in which the diagnosis seemed comparable to the type of injury suffered by the workers treated by the chiropractor, 41 percent of these workmen resumed work after one week of time-loss.

A study of time loss back claims, Workmen's Compensation Board, State of Oregon, March 1971.

EXHIBIT XX
New Zealand Royal Commission of Inquiry on Chiropractic

In 1979, a Royal Commission of Inquiry on Chiropractic in New Zealand, following an in-depth study concluded:

"The Commission has found it established beyond any reasonable degree of doubt that chiropractors have a more thorough training in spinal mechanics and spinal manual therapy than any other health professional. It would therefore be astonishing to contemplate that a chiropractor, in those areas of expertise, should be subject to the directions of a medical practitioner who is largely ignorant of those matter simply because he has had no training in them."

Inglis, BD, "Chiropractic in New Zealand: Report of the Commission of Inquiry into Chiropractic," Government Printer, Wellington, NZ, 1979.

EXHIBIT XXI
The Gallup Survey

A study by the Gallup Organization, reported in March 1991, was conducted to determine the attitudes, opinions and behaviors of both users and non-users of chiropractic services. Most of the 750 chiropractic users were last treated for a back and/or neck pain problem; 44 percent stating back pain/problem, 10 percent neck pain, 8 percent need adjustment, 7 percent accident/injury/fall, 4 percent muscle spasms/pains, 4 percent sciatica, 3 percent pinched nerve, 3 percent headaches, 3 percent shoulder pain, 3 percent ruptured disc, 2 percent arthritis, and 16 percent other.

Effectiveness outcomes: Overall, 90 percent felt that this treatment was effective, with 69 percent stating it was very effective and 21 percent reporting somewhat effective. More than 80 percent were satisfied with the treatment they received, with 61 percent being very satisfied and 23 percent somewhat satisfied. Nearly 75 percent felt that most of their expectations were met during the last visit or series of visits, 43 percent stating all expectations and 30 percent most expectations were met. Sixty-eight percent would likely see a doctor of chiropractic again for a treatment of a similar condition, with 47 percent stating that they definitely would and 21 percent stating that they probably would.

Outcomes: Nearly 80 percent of the chiropractic users felt that the cost of chiropractic treatment was reasonable, 38 percent said very reasonable and 40 percent somewhat reasonable.

Overall impression of doctors of chiropractic: On the average, chiropractic users rated doctors of chiropractic a "7" on a 10-point scale (10 = excellent); 50 percent rating them very good to excellent and 33 percent fair to good.

Gallup Organization, "Demographic Characteristics of Users of Chiropractic Services", Princeton, N.J., 1991.

EXHIBIT XXII
Lower Costs and Fewer Work Days Lost with Chiropractic Management in Australian Study

This retrospective Workers' Compensation study in Australia compared chiropractic and medical management of 1,996 cases of work-related mechanical low back pain. The number of compensation days taken by claimants was found to be significantly lower – an average of 6.26 days for chiropractic patients and 25.56 days for medical patients. The average cost of compensation was $392 for chiropractic management and $1,569 for medical management – four times greater than chiropractic costs.

Ebrall, PS, "Mechanical Low Back Pain: A Comparison of Medical and Chiropractic Management Within the Victorian WorkCare Scheme." *Chiropractic Journal of Australia,* June 1992, vol 22, #2, pp. 47-53.

ⒺⓍⒽⒾⒷⒾⓉ ⓍⓍⒾⒾⒾ
Improvement with Chiropractic Longer Lasting with Fewer Visits than Physical Therapy

This Dutch project compared the effectiveness of manipulation and physical therapy for the treatment of persistent back and neck complaints. The chiropractic treatment group showed greater improvement of the primary complaint, as well as improvement in physical function with fewer visits. It also demonstrated that manipulation and physical therapy are not interchangeable. The study concluded: Manipulative therapy and physiotherapy are better than general practitioner and placebo treatment. Furthermore, manipulative therapy is slightly better than physiotherapy after 12 months.

> Koes, BW, Bouter, LM et al., "Randomized Clinical Trial of Manipulative Therapy and Physiotherapy for Persistent Back and Neck Complaints: Results of One Year Follow Up, " *British Medical Journal*, 7 March 1992, vol 304, pp. 601-605.

ⒺⓍⒽⒾⒷⒾⓉ ⓍⒾⓋ
Manipulation of a Confirmed Disc Herniation

An article in *The Journal of Chiropractic Research and Clinical Investigation* (1992) by M. Siciliano, DC, T. Bernard, DC and N. Bentley, DC confirmed the reduction of a C5-C6 disc herniation. The case of a patient with a C5-C6 disc herniation, as documented by magnetic resonance imaging (MRI), is presented. The patient was rendered symptom-free after a series of manipulations of the cervical spine. A post-adjustment MRI, made following 13 adjustments, revealed that the herniation was reduced from its previously noted extent.

ⒺⓍⒽⒾⒷⒾⓉ ⓍⓍⓋ
The Most Effective Conservative Therapy in Whiplash Injuries

Researchers compared standard physical therapy methods to spinal manipulation in patients suffering from whiplash neck injuries. The study's main objective was to assess the long term effect of early mobilization exercises in patients with acute sprains of the neck after road accidents.

Results: Of the 167 patients responding, the percentage of patients still with symptoms was not significantly different in those receiving rest or physiotherapy (46 percent vs. 44 percent), but that in those receiving advice on early mobilization was significantly lower (23 percent).

Conclusions: Advice to mobilize in the early phase after neck injury reduces the number of patients with symptoms at two years and is superior to physiotherapy alone. Prolonged wearing of a collar is associated with persistence of symptoms.

> McKinney, LA. "Early mobilization and outcome in acute sprains of the neck," *British Medical Journal*, vol. 299, pp. 1006-8, 1989.

Medical vs. Chiropractic Costs

In one study, Dr. Stano et al. (1992) used the MEDSTAT systems database to develop a comprehensive database that would be suitable for research purposes, covering 2 million beneficiaries. The authors found that payments to chiropractors represent only 1.8 percent of total payments and "as a result would account for very little of the nation's rapid growth rates of health-care spending". Dr. Stano found that the cost per patient is lower for chiropractic care than for physician or osteopath care. For episodes lasting more than a day, the mean payment to DCs was $870 compared to $2,141 for MDs. Dr. Stano concluded that there is "little doubt that medical treatment for patients with comparable diagnostic codes is considerably more costly than chiropractic treatment."

Stano, M, Ehrhart, J. "The Growing Role of Chiropractic in Health Care Delivery. *"Journal of American Health Policy*, Nov/Dec 1992, vol 2, #6, pp. 39-45.

Savings from Chiropractic Care

One of the clearest statements on the cost-effectiveness of chiropractic care comes from the British trial (Meade et al., 1990). The committee declared that "the potential economic, resource and policy implications of our results are extensive." If patients with mechanical back pain were instead treated by chiropractors, the savings in health-care costs alone would be about $8 million annually. The reduction in time-loss would lead to further savings to industry of $26 million in output and another $6 million to government for reduced Social Security payments. The Committee stated:

> "There is economic support for use of chiropractic in low-back pain...consideration should be given to recognizing appropriately trained and experienced chiropractors and to providing chiropractic within the NHS, either in hospitals or by purchasing chiropractic treatment in existing clinics."

Meade T.W., Dyer S., et al. "Low Back Pain of Mechanical Origin: Randomized Comparison of Chiropractic and Hospital Outpatient Treatment." *British Medical Journal*, 2 June 1990, Vol 300 #67137, pp. 1431-1437.

Manual Therapy vs. Medical Care

A new controlled multicenter trial reveals manual therapy (spinal adjustments) is superior to conventional medical care in treating low back pain. One hundred-one outpatients with acute or subacute low back pain were randomly allocated to one of two treatment groups. One group received standard medical care by primary health-care teams. The other received manipulation, mobilization, muscle stretching, auto-traction and cortisone injections. The two groups were similar in most pre-trial variables. After one month of treatment, the proportion of patients on sick leave was six times larger in the conventionally treated group. Furthermore, by all measures, the group receiving specific manual treatment had a significantly better outcome.

Blomberg S, Swardsudd K, Mildenberger F. *The Journal of Othopaedic Medicine*, Vol 16, number one, 1994, pp. 2-8.

EXHIBIT XXIX
Exercise and Manipulation Provide Improvement

Patients with low back syndrome showed more rapid improvement with a combination of exercises and manipulation than with an established extension program alone. Twenty-four patients were randomly assigned to two groups. The first received an extension-oriented exercise and postural program, and the second received manipulation combined with a program of flexion and extension exercises. The second group received postero-lateral-inferior thrusts followed by hand-heel rocking. Following treatment, the authors concluded that "treating with a manipulative procedure directed toward the sacroiliac region, followed by an exercise program that includes both flexion and extension, results in more rapid resolution of symptoms and improvement in functional limitations than an established extension program alone."

Erhard RE, Delitto A, Cibulka MT. *Physical Therapy*, Vol 74, #12, December 1994, pp. 1094-1100.

EXHIBIT XXX
Disc Herniations Reduced by Chiropractic Adjustments.

Cervical and lumbar disc herniations are commonly encountered in clinical chiropractic practice. Clinical studies and case reports have addressed on the efficacy of chiropractic management for disc herniations. Imaging studies have shown disc resorption on follow-up CT or MRI subsequent to non-operative medical care. Of the 27 patients studied by repeat MRI, VAS and physical exam, 22 or 80 percent had a good clinical outcome. This consisted of reduced VAS scores below 2 and resolution of the patient's radicular pain. Seventeen of these 27 patients, or 63 percent, not only had a good clinical outcome but had evidence of resolution or reduction of disc herniations evident on repeat MRI.

BenEliyahu, DJ. "MRI Study of 27 Patients Receiving Chiropractic Treatment for Cervical and Lumbar Disc Herniations." A paper presented at the Conference Proceedings of the Chiropractic Centennial Foundation, Washington, DC, July, 1995.

⬚X⬚H⬚I⬚B⬚I⬚T ⬚X⬚X⬚X⬚I
Fifty-Year History of Chiropractic Effectiveness

Clinical trials published in the professional literature between 1930 and 1981 were examined in this report of the 18 randomized clinical trials that met the strict specifications of the Midwest Research Institute. On the basis of the studies, the report concluded: 1.) Manual therapy was superior to placebos; 2.) there was greater mobility following manipulation; 3.) the duration of treatment was shorter for manipulated groups; and 4.) there was improved lateral flexion and rotation after manipulation.

The report also concluded that, "...numerous case studies throughout the literature report the satisfaction of chiropractic patients with the outcome of treatments."

MacDonald, MJ, Morton, L. Chiropractic Evaluation Study Task III Report of the Relevant Literature, MRI Project No. 8533-D, For Department of Defense, OCHAMPUS, Aurora, Colorado, 24 January 1986.

⬚X⬚H⬚I⬚B⬚I⬚T ⬚X⬚X⬚X⬚I⬚I
Manga Report Summary on LBP

"In summary, with respect to the effectiveness of medical versus chiropractic management of LBP, the literature favors chiropractic. The literature is negative, inconclusive or virtually non-existent concerning many medical treatments, including the mainstay of bed rest if prolonged beyond two or three days. The many neutral to very positive findings on chiropractic manipulation, with no trial reporting ineffectiveness, presents a curious contrast full of irony. On the basis of the clinical research it is reasonable for private and public insurance managers to now call upon the medical profession to provide better evidence for the effectiveness of the standard therapies it uses. Yet, at present, it is the public perception due in part to medical criticism of chiropractic treatment as unscientific, that it is the chiropractors who have the most to prove concerning the efficacy and effectiveness of their therapeutic modalities. There is, for example, the thought-provoking claim from an eminent neurosurgeon in the U.S. that approximately 90 percent of the 250,000 back surgeries performed annually in that country could be avoided (Burton et al., 1992).

Policy Recommendations and Reform

"In our view, the constellation of the evidence of (a) the effectiveness and cost-effectiveness of chiropractic management of LBP, (b) untested, questionable and even harmful use of medical therapies by physicians, (c) the economic efficiency of chiropractic over physician care for LBP, (d) the safety of chiropractic care and (e) the preference and satisfaction expressed by patients of chiropractic, together offers an overwhelming case in favor of much greater use of chiropractic services for the management of LBP.

"However, the desired change in the health-care delivery system will not occur by itself, by accommodation between the professions, or by actions on the part of Workers' Compensation boards or the private sector generally. The government will have to instigate the reform and monitor the progress of the desired changes called for by our overall conclusion.

"There should be a shift in policy now to encourage the utilization of chiropractic services for the management of LBP, given the impressive body of evidence on the effectiveness and comparative cost-effectiveness of these services, and on the high levels of patient satisfaction.

"The shift in utilization from physician to chiropractic care should lead to significant savings in health-care expenditures judging from evidence in the Canada, the U.S., the U.K. and Australia, and even larger savings if a more comprehensive view of the economic costs of low back pain is taken.

"Unnecessary or failed surgery is not only wasteful and costly but, *ipso facto*, low quality medical care. The opportunity for consultations, second opinions and wider treatment options are significant advantages we foresee from this initiative which has been employed with success in a clinical research setting at the University Hospital, Saskatoon.

"A prominent medical organization, the North American Spine Society, has recently concluded that spinal manipulation, and specifically chiropractic adjustment, is an acceptable and effective treatment for most patients with lumbosacral disorders. This review, when coupled with more thorough analysis by prestigious institutions such as RAND Corporation, adds measurably to the growing credence in spinal manipulation as a therapy of choice for most low back pain."
Manga Pran, PhD, et al. "The Effectiveness and Cost-Effectiveness of Chiropractic Management of Low-Back Pain," Ontario Ministry of Health, 1993.

EXHIBITS OF PROOF
The Case Against Back Surgery

For too long the employers, lawyers, government officials and the general public have accepted the opinions of medical doctors as facts not to be challenged in matters of health-care. For instance, until recently the outdated concept that all back problems are due to disc abnormalities was considered "medical scripture" not to be questioned. Back surgeries were believed the only rational solution to back pain, and MDs ridiculed any other explanation or treatment. Together these mistaken beliefs have lead to an epidemic of back surgeries unparalleled in history.

The myopic medical mentality which professed drugs and surgery as the only solutions to all health problems has lead to an intransigence of progress unlike any other field. Indeed, if the electronics world was as slow to change, it would still be in the vacuum tube era instead of microchips! Consequently, many medical methods have avoided the scrutiny and rigors of open competition that all other fields have faced. The result has been many outdated, ineffective and costly medical treatments that have lead to a huge crisis in clinical effectiveness, as well as cost-effectiveness.

The Manga Report discussed the consequences of this medical intransigence in regard to the epidemic of back problems:

> "It is widely known that about 70 percent or more of existing medical technology and procedures have not been subjected to adequate cost-effectiveness analysis... Some of these developments are concerned mainly with questions of efficacy, while others have a more extended concern and include questions of cost-effectiveness....There is no question that many of these studies are motivated by concerns about the very sizeable cost and the economic waste of inappropriate care... At least 30 percent of hospital admissions are thought to be inappropriate.... Other concerns are the quality of care, and the desire by patients and public generally for more informed decisions about health-care treatment."

It is well known that the current managed health-care programs such as Worker's Compensation and many personal injury cases are still troubled by high costs and clinically ineffective methods for spinal treatment. Although chiropractic care is included in state and federal Workers' Compensation programs, the "system" still relies heavily on medical analysis and treatment for spinal injuries. For personal injury/auto accident cases, too many attorneys still rely on their medical friends for the management of these cases, despite the overwhelming evidence that proves chiropractic management is best for the vast majority of spinal injuries. Unfortunately, the higher medical costs from ineffective surgery and treatments may actually be an incentive for both surgeons and for attorneys who seek higher settlements due to larger medical expenses.

No reform will occur as long as the principals are prospering financially. The medical profession has no interest in doing less surgery as long as the lucrative fees exist. Many attorneys have little interest in referring patients to chiropractors if it will mean a lower settlement. The Manga Report mentions this dilemma:

"The role of medicine in this work will be significant but it must not dominate: After all it is due to the absence of scientific rigor in medicine that we are so ignorant about appropriateness and cost-effectiveness today!

"The boundaries between health-care professions have and will continue to change because of the changes in educational systems, medical technologies, information systems, insurance coverage, and the organization of health-care services. Keeping service boundaries intact is an illusory and unwise goal and is counterproductive to the objective of improving the efficiency of our health-care system. Turf is money – it is important to understand that battles over professional turf will shape to a considerable extent the nature and design of the new health-care system. Suffice it to say, there is great scope for professions other than medical doctors to assume greater responsibilities in delivering services and caring for patients..."

Let the following research studies prove to you the facts against back surgery. You might be surprised to learn of the overwhelming arguments against this radical, ineffective and expensive form of back treatment. Let the experts convince you, as they have convinced researchers like Dr. Manga and the expert panel of the AHCPR, to name but a few of the many investigators who have concluded that spinal manipulation is in and back surgeries are out.

EXHIBIT XXXIII
"Ruptured Discs Not Always A Pain"
Research suggests too much emphasis is placed on them
Associated Press Article

"Boston – Ruptured discs, long considered the hallmark of a bad back, are so common among perfectly pain-free people that some question whether doctors should try so hard to find them.

A study being published found that about a quarter of people with no history of back trouble whatsoever have ruptured discs when examined with magnetic resonance imaging scans, or MRIs.

The research suggests that ruptured discs may not mean much for many people, and they certainly cannot be assumed to be the source of a patient's backache.

The study, conducted by radiologists, also casts doubt on wide use of one of the mainstays of their profession – employing MRIs to look for quirks in the lower spine.

With MRIs so widely available, many doctors now routinely order them as a first step when they see patients with back problems. If they find a bad-looking disc – what is commonly called a ruptured or herniated disc or disc prolapse – they may send patients on for a more invasive test called discography. After that may come surgery.

The study suggests that disc peculiarities "may frequently be coincidental" in people with back trouble. In other words, the disc might not be the cause of the pain. And if so, fixing it is a waste.

The study was conducted on 98 healthy volunteers by Dr. Maureen C. Jensen and colleagues from Hoag Memorial Hospital in Newport Beach, Calif. The work, published in *The New England Journal of Medicine*, roughly duplicates a study completed four years ago by Dr. Scott Boden, an orthopedic surgeon at Emory University.

'The MRI should never be used as a screening test, which is unfortunately the way it is very commonly used today,' Boden said. 'In fact, use of the MRI too early in somebody's disease process can result in seeing these findings that are like gray hair – everybody gets them – and can result in over-treatment.'

In other studies, Boden has also found that MRIs can spot disc degeneration in people with fine-feeling necks, as well as torn cartilage in those with pain-free knees.

Backache is one of the most common miseries of adulthood. An estimated 31 million American complain of low back pain at any given time. It is also one of the most costly ailments, accounting for $8 billion in medical care annually.

EXHIBIT XXXIV
The Placebo Effects of Back Surgery

Researchers are well aware of the placebo effect in health care treatments. The common belief is that one-third of patients will recover from a condition after receiving a "sham" treatment, rather than the real thing. An article in the *JAMA* discusses the placebo effect with back surgery. This article reiterates that it is unclear what real value, if any, surgery holds for patients with back pain.

"Placebo effects of back surgery are suggested by Spangfort's review of long-term outcomes of 2,504 diskectomies for lumbar disk disease. Complete relief of sciatica was noted in 37% and complete relief of back pain in 43% of patients who had no disk herniation. There is no known therapeutic effect of surgical exploration of the lumbar spine, changes in patient status were most likely attributable to placebo effect and natural history.

"The success rates after sham or discredited procedures may be compared to the success rates in spine surgery case series. Across 74 studies of surgery for lumbar spinal stenosis, an average of 64% of patients had good or excellent outcomes. Similarly, 68% of patients had good or excellent results among 47 studies of lumbar spinal fusions. These figures reflect outcomes reported at long-term follow-up; the absence of randomized controlled trials precludes the interpretation of the outcomes as resulting from specific surgery effects plus natural history. However, the figures are similar to the average 70% excellent or good outcomes for several abandoned medical and surgical therapies.

"In sum, nonspecific influences plus natural history and regression to the mean play an important role in pain relief after surgery. Important nonspecific influences likely include subjects' and surgeons' expectations of improvement.

This situation with respect to low back surgery is highlighted further by the weak association between imaging test results and symptoms, and between technical success of surgery (e.g., solid fusion) and symptom improvement."

Turner et al. The importance of placebo effects in pain treatment and research. *JAMA* 1994;271:1609-1614.

🄴🅇🄷🄸🄱🄸🅃 🅇🅇🅇🅅
Keynote Neurosurgeon Blasts Medical Approach

Hubert Rosomoff, MD, neurosurgeon at the University of Miami, after 15 years of surgery on several thousand patients with back and leg pain, decided that, "Disc herniation, even when clearly visible through imaging, was seldom the real cause of pain...and that 99 percent of back pain patients didn't need surgery... Back pain should be viewed as a non-surgical problem, subject to few exceptions."

His extensive non-surgical experience has convinced him that:

"A simple medical back examination is no good...the underlying problem is usually missed...all chronic low-back pain is an iatrogenic disability because of unskilled diagnosis and management...the herniated disc doesn't produce pain *per se*...there is no evidence that muscle relaxants will help mechanical contraction of muscle."

The Chiropractic Report, July 1988 vol. 2, no. 5, editor David Chapman-Smith, LLB.

🄴🅇🄷🄸🄱🄸🅃 🅇🅇🅇🅅🄸
The High Costs of Spinal Surgery

The costs of the 500,000 back surgeries done each year add up quickly.

1.) Surgeon's fees alone may cost from $5,600 for a discectomy to $12,500 for a fusion.

2.) Hospital fees may run from $12,000 to $15,000, depending upon the length of stay, notwithstanding any additional costs from complication.

3.) Rehabilitation costs may be hundreds of dollars per day up to 12 months of rehab.

4.) Medication, psychological therapy, lost wages and possible disability costs all add to the final cost of a single back surgery.

5.) Approximately 40 percent of these patients return for a second surgery due to recurring pain.

6.) Considering that 90 percent of these surgeries are deemed unnecessary or ineffective; there is a huge savings to be made by finding more effective treatments and methods of prevention – the chiropractic solution.

7.) In 1985 U.S. Workers' Compensations boards disbursed $6 billion for low back pain.

8.) Some estimates claim that 10 times more back surgeries occur in the U.S. than in any other country.

9.) No one knows the true cost, and as the manager of a large insurance association confessed, "The insurance industry should be and is being criticized for an obvious lack of statistical data on the costs of back-related injuries. What we have, however, is scary."

Anonymous (1990) "Low back pain: the scorecard," *Harvard Medical School Health Letter*, vol. 15, no. 11, pp. 1-3.

⊞⊠ℍ𝕀𝔹𝕀𝕋 ⊠⊠⊠𝕍𝕀𝕀
The Costs Associated with Back Surgery

The high costs of medical management of low back pain is a major subject in the scientific literature in recent years. In a 1987 report by Dr. G. Waddell, titled "A New Clinical Model for the Treatment of Low Back Pain," which also won the 1987 Volvo Prize for spinal clinical research, revealed startling results that shocked the medical establishment:

1.) Surgery and chemonucleolysis have been subject to high failure rates and unacceptable costs and are now used rarely, with under 1 percent of patients.

2.) Bed rest, which promotes "illness behavior" and the huge compensation costs has now been proved ineffective. It has been a general medical first response to back pain, along with pain pills and muscle relaxants, none of which have proven to be clinically effective.

3.) The basic approach to treatment now recommended is the chiropractic model – early active treatment (spinal manipulations) to restore spinal joint function and to prevent the onset of bed rest illness behavior.

4.) Chiropractic spinal care has proven effective; and it produces a generally quick response and is also cost-effective, both in terms of direct costs (treatments) and indirect costs (compensation, lost production, lost wages, etc.).

Waddell, G. "A New Clinical Model for the Treatment of Low Back Pain." Spine 12(7): 632-644.

⊞⊠ℍ𝕀𝔹𝕀𝕋 ⊠⊠⊠𝕍𝕀𝕀𝕀
The Controversy of Back Surgery
Journal of the American Medical Association

According to a study reported in *JAMA* (August 1992) titled "Patient Outcomes After Lumbar Spinal Fusions," the medical investigators stunned their colleagues with the announcement that:

"For several low back disorders, no advantage has been demonstrated for fusion over surgery without fusion...Complications of fusions are common...

"The role of spinal fusion in the treatment of many lumbar spine disorders remains controversial...Even greater controversy surrounds the indications for fusion in patients with degenerative spondylolisthesis, degenerative disc disease, or failed back surgery syndrome...

"Other concerns are the poor association sometimes found between fusion and pain relief...

122

"Despite these uncertainties and problems, fusions were performed at
a steadily increasing rate in the U.S. from 1979 through 1987."
This study indicates that only 16 percent of fusion patients report satisfactory results and that the complications from spinal surgeries oftentime are as problematic as the back pain itself. Some of the reported complications included: mortality, paralysis, deep infection, superficial infection, thrombosis, embolus, neural injury, donor site infection, chronic pain, pelvic instability, graft extrusion, substance abuse, psychological risks and depression, and 8 percent of fused patients required subsequent surgery to remove additional disc material.

"Because the literature does not establish the usefulness of fusion for
the conditions we have reviewed, and because fusion is associated
with significant costs and complications, such research should have a
high priority," according to the *JAMA* authors.

ⒺⓍⒽⒾⒷⒾⓉ ⓍⓍⓍⒾⓍ
Lumbar Fusion Not Effective

This study by G.M. Franklin, MD, was designed to produce clear clinical results for lumbar fusion in injured workers. The results indicate that more than two-thirds of lumbar fusion patients (68 percent) were still totally work-disabled two years after surgery. These findings are in contrast to previous reports indicating a satisfactory outcome in an average of 68 percent of cases. Further, fixation devices like pedicle screws were found to increase the likelihood of re-operation after lumbar fusion. The study also found, "most patients reported that back pain (67.7 percent) was worse and overall quality of life (55.8 percent) was no better or worse than before surgery. Outcome of lumbar fusion performed on injured workers was worse than reported in published case series."

Franklin GM, et al., *Spine*, vol 19 #17, Sept. 1, 1994, pp. 1897-1903.

ⒺⓍⒽⒾⒷⒾⓉ ⓍⓍⓍⓍ
"Low Back Pain and Sciatica."
Journal of the American Medical Association

In May 1967 the AMA was told by John C. Wilson, Jr., MD, chairman of the AMA's section on orthopedic surgery, and later, president of the American Academy of Orthopedic Surgeons, that medical doctors and orthopedic surgeons were essentially ignorant of the causes or corrections of low back problems.

Dr. Wilson concluded that:

1.) Patients were operated upon after inadequate evaluations.

2.) There was too much reliance by physicians on poor quality x-ray films.

3.) Surgery was often done only because of an abnormality in a myelogram without reference to plain films of the lower spine.

4.) Exploratory surgery upon the lower back was done without sufficient clinical basis.

5.) Extensive surgery was often done for solely subjective complaints.

6.) Repeated attempts at spinal fusion – sometimes six or eight tries -
- were often performed by surgeons of limited experience.

7.) Surgery was often authorized by industrial accident commissions comprised exclusively of laymen.

8.) Extensive removal of posterior vertebral elements by neurosurgeons made stabilization of the lower portion of the spine technically difficult if not impossible.

🄴🅇🄷🄸🄱🄸🅃 🅇🅇🅇🅇🄸
Manga Report

In this extensive study of LBP, the researchers commented on surgical interventions:

1.) "Surgery should be considered only when conservative treatment modalities have failed to reverse significant functional impairment... As new and more effective methods of conservative treatments are introduced, the need for surgery decreases... An important point to be made here is that there is very little consensus within the medical community on the appropriateness and efficacy of performing surgery for LBP."

2.) "Chemonucleolysis: This Task Force concluded that this treatment is not useful in recurring LBP, and can in fact be contra-indicated if a first injection fails."

3.) "Spinal Fusion: Fusion surgery is inherently more complicated, more painful, and riskier than procedures such as discectomy and laminectomy. Even when the operation goes well, the patient spends over a week in the hospital and requires a recuperation period of several months."

4.) "Lumbar Laminectomy: A standard lumbar laminectomy is quite uncomfortable, requiring average hospitalizations in excess of five days. Rehabilitation is often delayed by postoperative discomfort."

5.) "Discectomy: This operation must be reserved for patients with a proven discal hernia who have not responded to conservative treatment."

Manga Pran, PhD, et al., "The Effectiveness and Cost-Effectiveness of Chiropractic Management of Low-Back Pain," Ontario Ministry of Health, 1993.

🄴🅇🄷🄸🄱🄸🅃 🅇🅇🅇🅇🄸🄸
Hospitals Waste Nearly $1 Billion on Low-Back Pain Treatment New Study Reports 78 percent of Hospital Days for Medical Back Problems Inappropriate.

Spine magazine featured the paper, "Nonsurgical Hospitalization for Low-Back Pain: Is It Necessary?" Authors Dr. Daniel Cherkin and Dr. Richard Deyo analyzed three sources of data for the hospitalization and care of low back pain patients in the state of Washington. Both authors are part of the back pain outcomes assessment team for the Agency of Health Care Policy and Research, with Dr. Deyo acting as principal investigator. They state:

"The picture that emerges is consistent with the other published analyses of the appropriateness of hospitalizations for medical back problems, which suggested that 70 percent of hospitalizations and 80 percent of hospital days were inappropriate...

"At the 1989 average hospital cost of $637 per day this would represent for a single year almost one billion dollars in unnecessary hospital expenses alone...

"The study also noted that CT scans, MRIs and other costly diagnostic tests probably incurred unnecessary hospitalization. Various forms of treatment including epidural steroid injections and bed rest also included unnecessary inpatient care."

EXHIBIT XXXXIII
Experts Criticize Medical Treatments for LBP

According to Dr. G. Waddell in his article that appeared in *Spine* magazine in 1987, "Modern medicine can successfully treat many serious spinal diseases and persisting nerve compression but has completely failed to cure the vast majority of patients with simple low-back pain. Over-emphasis of pain alone, over-dependence on a nominal diagnosis of disc prolapse, and over-prescription of rest may indeed be a major cause of iatrogenic disability."

According to Dr. R.A. Deyo in his 1983 article in *JAMA*, "...very relevant questions that ...medical care ought to answer are just 'how and why do so many medical technologies and procedures used in the medical management of LBP get adopted and diffused so widely without clinical evidence of their effectiveness?' Dr. Deyo concluded in his investigation of medical therapies for LBP that "there was no convincing evidence to support the efficacy of corsets, bed rest, TENS, conventional traction or drug use."

Another review concluded, "that prolonged rest and passive physical therapy modalities no longer have a place in the treatment of the chronic problem of LBP." (Mooney, 1987).

There is certainly more scientific evidence in support of the use of early exercise than for passive physical therapies, according to a 1992 study by Dr. Deyo. It is also quite clear that the evidence on the effectiveness of exercise is not as strong as that for manipulation. It seems reasonable to conclude on the basis of the present literature that management of most patients with LBP should include manipulation and the use of early exercises.

Waddell, G. "A new clinical model for the treatment of low back pain." *Spine*, vol. 12, no. 7, pp. 632-644. 1987.

Deyo, RA. "Conservative therapy for low back pain: distinguishing useful from useless therapy." *JAMA*, vol. 250, no. 8, pp. 1057-1063. 1983.

Mooney, V. "Where is the pain coming from?" *Spine*, vol. 12. no. 8, pp. 754-759. 1987.

EXHIBIT XXXXIV
Spinal Fusions Questioned

The use of spinal fusion as a treatment for LBP has gained prominence in recent years and has sparked much controversy. In a review of the literature to assess the efficacy of spinal fusions in the management of LBP, no randomized trials were identified, and the authors concluded that, "for several low-back disorders no advantage has been demonstrated for fusion over surgery without fusion, and complications of fusions are common" (Turner et al. 1992).

Over a seven year period, O'Beirne et al., in 1992 found that there was no correlation between success or failure of the fusion and relief of pain, which suggests that patients gained relief from the 'natural history of the underlying condition' rather than the operation. Dr. Deyo (1992) cautioned that patients who had fusions had worse outcomes than patients who didn't have fusions. He stated that, "in fusion cases, the rate of in-hospital complications was nearly twice as great and post-operative mortality was nearly four times as high, and the likelihood of blood transfusion was nearly four times as high... And the fusion operations didn't reduce the subsequent likelihood of reoperation or rehospitalization for back pain."

O'Beirne J, O'Neill D, Gallagher J, et al. "Spinal fusion for back pain: a clinical and radiographic review." *J. Spinal Dis* 5(1):32-28, 1992.

EXHIBIT XXXXV
Informed Consent in Washington State

In the *State Provider Update*, Volume I, number 7, January 1995, the state of Washington mandated that before any worker consents to a lumbar fusion, the following form titled, "Lumbar Fusion Patient Consent Form" must be signed and sent to the state:

"As part of the Department's utilization management program, guidelines for various surgical procedures have been developed. The guidelines for lumbar fusion require that you be aware of the following. Please review the items below, with your physician, and sign (indicating that you understand and that you still wish to proceed with the fusion).

"The chances of an injured worker being off disability two years after fusion are only 23 percent. More than 50 percent of workers who received lumbar fusion, in Washington Worker's Compensation, felt that both pain and functional recovery were no better or worse after lumbar fusion.

"Pain relief, even when present, is not likely to be complete.

"The overall rate of re-operation within two years, for all fusions, is approximately 23 percent. The use of instrumentation in Washington workers nearly doubled the risk of re-operation.

"Pedicle screw devices are NOT approved for use in the spine by the FDA."

126

Conclusion: The Debate Is Over!

The scientific debate is over and chiropractic clearly has won. Not only did the AHCPR's two-year review of 4,000 articles about back pain from the Library of Congress endorse spinal manipulation over all medical methods, but additional research has emerged from other countries which agrees and also endorses chiropractic care for back pain. The British Research Council completed a 10-year study on back pain and concluded that chiropractic care is twice as effective as anything medicine had to offer. The Ontario Ministry of Health's Manga Report conducted an extensive investigation into back problems and also endorsed chiropractic as the safest and most effective treatment. Numerous state Workers' Compensation studies in the U.S. have also looked into this expensive problem and all have concluded that chiropractic care is the most clinically and cost-effective means of care. The unbiased international research has clearly proven that for the vast majority of back problems, spinal manipulation is superior to the medical management for low back pain.

If anyone – your MD, DO, PT, attorney, teacher, mother, father, sister or brother – tries to convince you otherwise, you must simply understand you're listening to someone terribly uninformed. Don't let the outdated "conventional wisdom" of the medical world deter you from the whole truth on this important matter. Don't let *voo-doo* surgeons scare you into ineffective (but profitable) back surgeries. Don't be fooled by MRI exams which show nice little pictures of disc problems which, in reality, may have nothing to do with your back pain. And most of all, don't fall prey to medical bigotry that speaks negatively about chiropractic care. The debate is over and the results emphatically state: Chiropractic is the best care for the vast majority of back attacks.

Unfortunately, too many people have been victimized by improper, unproven and ineffective medical procedures like pain pills, muscle relaxants, injections, hot packs, ultrasound, traction and, worst of all, back surgeries. Not only have too many people suffered from these ineffective medical treatments, too many people still suffer from the medical bigotry accumulated through decades of a well-orchestrated propaganda campaign against chiropractic. This propaganda led to a federal judge's injunction in 1987 against the AMA's antitrust behavior, even going so far as to criticize the AMA's actions as complete "lawlessness." This illegal and unethical campaign to discredit chiropractic in the mind of the public has lead to an epidemic of back problems unparalleled in the world. Not only have chiropractors been the victims of this propaganda, so too have been the generations of Americans who believed these lies and have suffered the consequences of unnecessary back surgeries or decided to "live with pain" because chiropractic care was disavowed in their minds as a possible solution.

I believe before any scientific proof about the effectiveness of chiropractic care will convince you or anyone else, we must start with a clean slate on this matter. Forget about the medical propaganda that you've heard from medical bigots. Forget about the "conventional wisdom" espoused by your medical doctors. Forget about the hearsay you've heard from your uninformed neighbors. Forget about the embellished scare stories in the media. Instead, I suggest you listen to the experts who have researched this issue and have accepted and supported the superiority of chiropractic spinal care. Listen to patients who have experienced firsthand the benefits of spinal adjustments. Listen to the medical failures who have still responded to chiropractic care despite their failed back surgeries. I urge you to make an informed decision about this important, pervasive problem that will affect most people sometime in their lives.

Keep in mind Her Majesty's Stationary Office in London in its *Report of a Clinical Standards Advisory Group Committee on Back Pain* which clearly stated: "Traditional medical treatment has failed to halt this epidemic and may even have contributed to it. There is a clear need to reconsider our whole approach to the management of low back pain and disability." If a conservative government in England can open its mind to reconsideration of this massive problem, I might add it's time for people everywhere to reconsider their present attitudes about spinal care before more of them suffer needlessly from ineffective drugs and back surgeries. Indeed, it's time for everyone to "think out of the medical box" of solutions to back pain.

The evidence is proof-positive. Chiropractic spinal care not only has passed the scrutiny of international researchers, it has been proven to be twice as effective clinically in returning patients to work. Further, studies have proven the cost-effectiveness of chiropractic care over the medical management of spinal problems of similar conditions. No longer can anyone question chiropractic's overall effectiveness. The facts are clear, and chiropractic, to the surprise of most everyone, has come out on top! As the Manga Report researchers stated: "Spinal manipulation applied by chiropractors is shown to be more effective than alternative [medical] treatments for LBP... There is an overwhelming body of evidence indicating that chiropractic management of low-back pain is more cost-effective than medical management."

Despite historical resistance by some medical physicians and despite economic disincentives such as a lack of insurance coverage, the public has long supported chiropractic care. Even the biased study by Dr. Tim Carey from the North Carolina Back Pain Project concluded that "Patients who saw chiropractors reported a significantly higher degree of satisfaction than those who saw practitioners in the other four strata." Drs. Cherkin and MacCornack found that patients' satisfaction with DCs was triple that of MDs! The utilization of chiropractic and other alternative health care methods has grown everywhere despite the private out-of-pocket costs to patients, mainly because these methods are effective. As with any product or service, the true test of viability rests in the marketplace – if it doesn't work, the consumer won't buy it. I dare say that if these expensive and ineffective back surgeries were not artificially supported by health insurance in the sham marketplace of health care, these cost-prohibitive procedures would have disappeared long ago. How many patients can afford a $14,000 back surgery that has such a low rate of success? Few, indeed!

In Canada, respondents gave the lowest score to physicians for the treatment of back pain. According to the Manga Report: "This is a clear message that the public in British Columbia does not believe that *medical* management of LBP is effective. The contrast could hardly have been more marked...Chiropractic meets the market test of consumer choice and preference. Simply put, despite economic disincentives for use of chiropractic services, chiropractic has met the market test of consumer choice and preference." Can you imagine the incredible benefits more people would enjoy if chiropractic care had equal coverage in every health program in every country? The potential to reduce costs and suffering would be immense!

Obviously, the solution to the management of back pain, the second largest cause of disability in our country, is the shift from medical to chiropractic management. The facts from a wide body of evidence from around the world have proven repeatedly the benefits of chiropractic care. Again, the Manga Report suggests: "There would be highly significant cost savings if more management of LBP was transferred from physicians to chiropractors. Evidence from Canada and other countries suggests potential savings of many hundreds of millions annually." As the Health Care Reform matures and managed care organizations strive to contain costs, this area of back surgeries is clearly one where millions, nay billions, of dollars could be saved.

Unfortunately, as the awareness about the effectiveness of spinal manipulation continues to grow, some imposters have already made efforts to misinform the public as to the real experts in this area. Don't be fooled by PTs or MDs who naively attempt the art of spinal adjustments. Again, recall the research which indicated that manipulation by chiropractors was superior to manipulation done by non-DCs. The New Zealand Commission of Inquiry into Chiropractic "found that no other health professional was as well qualified to carry out a diagnosis for spinal dysfunction or to perform manipulation therapy." Indeed, consumer beware!

There you have it – the facts are clear that chiropractic works faster, cheaper, better and safer, and more proof that medical management is quite risky, clinically-ineffective and costly. So, the next time you or someone in your family has a back attack, keep in mind these facts. The 20th century disaster of low back pain has a good solution, but one the medical establishment has long fought to deny to the public. Unless this medical obstructionist attitude ceases, this 20th century disaster will certainly become a 21st century disaster as well. Until the public understands this irrational source of skepticism toward chiropractors, back problems will continue to plague our society. The sooner you and your family incorporate chiropractic spinal care into your family's health regimen, just as you have dental care, the sooner you will avoid the tragedy of disabling low back pain, scoliosis development, neck pains and headaches.

As a practicing chiropractor, I would be amiss if I failed to mention that you don't need just a back attack to see a chiropractor. While this research focused primarily on chiropractic's effectiveness with back pain, more research currently is being conducted on the chiropractic management of other common health problems such as asthma, hypertension, infantile colic, otitis media, enuresis, scoliosis, migraine headaches, dysmenorrhea, PMS, and carpal tunnel syndrome, to name just a few.

I believe that the more the scientific community learns about the clinical effectiveness of chiropractic care, the more it will come to the conclusion which chiropractors have long known: That chiropractic works for many problems, not just back pain. Although this belief remains a controversial issue to the uninformed who don't understand the concept of neuro-physiology in health care, it remains the salient principle of the chiropractic profession – its Big Idea of health care. However, that concept is another book altogether, but it is a lesson you can learn for yourself by visiting your local chiropractor's office. He or she will be glad to teach you that inside the spinal column is the incredible nerve system that commands and controls every function in your body. You will then understand not only that chiropractic is best for spinal problems, but you will discover how chiropractic care can help you and your family stay well, naturally.

But, in regard to this epidemic of back pain, there is one absolutely indisputable message: Chiropractic is the best treatment for the vast majority of back pain cases. If your goal is to avoid a back surgery, I suggest you consider using chiropractic care – the *proven* method for back pain.

References

Chapter One

1. Pran Manga, PhD, et al., "The Effectiveness and Cost-Effectiveness of Chiropractic Management of Low-Back Pain," Ontario Ministry of Health, 1993.

2. M.C. Jensen et al., "Magnetic Resonance Imaging of the Lumbar Spine in People Without Back Pain," *The New England Journal of Medicine* 331(2):60-73 (1994).

3. S.D. Boden et al., "Abnormal Magnetic-Resonance Scans of the Lumbar Spine in Asymptomatic Subjects," *J. Bone Joint Surgery (AM)* 72(3):403-8 (1990).

4. B.E. Finneson, "A Lumbar Disc Surgery Predictive Score Card: A Retrospective Evaluation," *Spine* (1979): 141-144.

5. W.H. Kirkaldy-Willis and D. Cassidy, Can. Fam. Phys. 31 (1985)::535-40.

6. N. Bogduk, "Clinical Anatomy of the Lumbar Spine," pp. 170.

7. V. Mooney, Spine 12(6):754-59 (1987).

8. P.G. Shekelle et al., "The Appropriateness of Spinal Manipulation for Low-Back Pain," RAND Corporation Report, 1992.

9. D.C. Cherkin and F.A. MacCornack, "Patient Evaluation of Low Back Pain Care from Family Physicians and Chiropractors" *West. J. Med.*, 150 (March 1989):351-355.

10. S. Bigos, O. Bowyer, G. Braen et al., "Acute Low Back Problems in Adults, Clinical Practice Guideline No. 14," Public Health Service, U.S. Department of Health and Human Services, AHCPR Publication No. 95-0642. Rockville, MD: December 1994.

Chapter Two

1. Earl Ubell, "What Works Best for Back Pain," *Parade Magazine* (Jan. 14, 1996): 12-13.

2. A.C. Papageorpiou et al., "Estimating the prevalence of low back pain in the general population," *Spine* (1995) 20: 1889-1894.

3. Ubell, ibid.

4. Ubell, ibid.

5. Margaret Mushinski, "Average Hospital Charges for Medical and Surgical Treatment of Back Problems: United States, 1993," *Statistical Bulletin*, (April-June 1995): Metropolitan Life Insurance Company, Health and Safety Education Division, Medical Department.

6. B.S. Webster and S.H. Snook, *Spine,* 19(10): 1111-1116 (1994).

7. G. Waddell, "Modern Management of Spinal Disorders," Conference proceedings of the Chiropractic Centennial Foundation, July 6-8, 1995, 169-180.

8. Pran Manga et al., "Chiropractic Management."

9. M. Rosen, A. Breen et al. "Management Guidelines for Back Pain Appendix B in Report of a Clinical Standards Advisory Group Committee on Back Pain," Her Majesty's Stationery Office, London 1994.

10. D. M. Eisenberg et al., "Unconventional Medicine in the United States," *New England Journal of Medicine*, 328(4): 246-252 (January 28, 1993).

11. C. Hawk, L.Z. Killinger, and M.E. Dusio, "Perceived Barriers to Chiropractic Utilization: Qualitative Study Using Focus Groups," *Journal of the American Chiropractic Association*, 32(6): 39-44 (1995).

12. P. Joseph Lisa, *The Assault on Medical Freedom*, (Norfolk, Va.: Hamptoms Road, 1994).

13. Sue A. Blevins, "The Medical Monopoly: Protecting Consumers or Limiting Competition?" *Policy Analysis,* Cato Institute, Washington, DC., (Dec. 15, 1995).

14. Julian Whitaker, "Health & Healing," newsletter, 4(11): November, 1994.

15. B.D. Inglis, "Chiropractic in New Zealand: Report of the Commission of Inquiry into

Chiropractic," Wellington, New Zealand, Government Printer, 1979.

16. D.C. Cherkin and F.A. MacCornack, "Patient Evaluation."

17. Gallup Organization, "Demographic Characteristics of Users of Chiropractic Services," Princeton, N.J., 1991.

18. W.B. Parsons and H.K. Boake, "Manipulation for Backache and Sciatica," *Journal Applied Therapeutics,* November 1966.

19. *Wilk v. AMA* U.S. District Court, Northern District of Illinois, September 25, 1987.

20. *Ibid,* May 6, 1987.

21. D.C. Cherkin, F.A. MacCornack, A.O. Berg, "Managing Low Back Pain – A Comparison of the Beliefs and Behaviours of Family Physicians and Chiropractors. *Western Journal of Medicine.* 149(4): 475-80 (1988).

22. D.C. Cherkin and F.A. MacCornack, "Patient Evaluation."

23. P. Joseph Lisa, *The Assault on Medical Freedom,* (Norfolk, Va.: Hamptoms Road, 1994).

24. Lynn Payer, *Disease-Mongers,* (John Wiley & Sons, 1992).

Chapter Three

1. S. Bigos et al., "Acute Low Back Problems in Adults," AHCPR Clinical Practice Guideline.

2. *Ibid.*

3. S. Bigos et al., "Understanding Acute Low Back Problems," "Acute Low Back Problems in Adults, Quick Reference Guide, No. 14," Public Health Service, U.S. Department of Health and Human Services, AHCPR Publication No. 95-0642, Rockville, MD: December 1994.

4. Pran Manga et al., "Chiropractic Management."

5. T.W. Meade et al., "Low Back Pain of Mechanical Origin; Randomized Comparison of Chiropractic and Hospital Outpatient Treatment," *BMJ* 300 (1990):1431-37.

6. Lee Casey, "Challenges of the Spine Specialists," *Spine* 20 (16): 1749-1752 (1994).

7. D.C. Cherkin et al., "An International Comparison of Back Surgery Rates," *Spine* 19 (11): 1201-1206 (1994).

8. H. Davis, "Increasing Rate of Cervical and Lumbar Spine Surgery in the United States, 1979-1990," *Spine* 19 (10): 1117-1124 (1994).

9. Ruth Jackson, *The Cervical Syndrome,* 4th ed. (Charles C. Thomas, Publisher; Springfield, Illinois, 1977).

10. *Ibid.*

11. D.C. Cherkin et al., "International Comparison."

12. G. Waddell and O.B. Allan, "A Historical Perspective on Low Back Pain and Disability," *Acta Orthop Scand* 60 (Suppl 234), 1989.

13. *Ibid.*

14. G. Waddell, "Modern Management of Spinal Disorders," presented at the Chiropractic Centennial Foundation, Washington, DC, 1995.

15. R.A. Deyo, "Back Pain: Best Treatment is Surprisingly Simple," *Consumer Reports,* September 1995.

16. Arthur Croft and Stephen Foreman, *Whiplash Injuries - The Cervical Acceleration/ Deceleration Syndrome,* (Baltimore: Williams & Wilkins, 1988.)

17. Lynn Payer, *Disease-Mongers,* (John Wiley & Sons, 1992.)

18. B. Rydevik, Department of Orthopaedics, University of Gothenburg, Sweden.

19. P.R. Luers, "Lumbosacral Spine Imaging: Physioanatomic Method," *Curr. Probl. Diagn. Radiol.,* 21 (5): 151-213, Sep-Oct 1992, Dept. of Radiology, Univ. of Utah Med. Center, Salt Lake City.

20. D. Borenstein, "Epidemiology, Etiology, Diagnostic Evaluation, and Treatment of Low Back Pain," *Curr. Opin. Rheumatol.* Mar 1995, 7 (2): 141-6, George Washington University

Medical Center, Washington, DC.

21. H.R. Grable, "Abnormal Findings on Magnetic Resonance Imaging in a Group of Motor Vehicle Accident Patients with Low Back Pain," *Am. J. Med. Qual.* Winter 1993, 8 (4): 194-96.

22. K.B. Wood et al., "Magnetic Resonance Imaging of the Thoracic Spine: Evaluation of Asymptomatic Individuals," Dept Orthopaedic Surgery, University of Minnesota. *J. Bone Joint Surgery* Nov. 1995, 77 (11): 1631-38.

23. W.O. Spitzer et al., "Redefining Whiplash and its Management," Quebec Task Force on Whiplash-Associated Disorders, May 1995.

24. R.A. Deyo, "Conservative Therapy for Low Back Pain - Distinguishing Useful From Useless Therapy," *JAMA* (1983) 250:1057-1062.

25. W.P. Butt, St. James' University Hospital, *British Journal of Rheumatology.*

26. S. Bigos, "Acute Problems in Adults," AHCPR Clinical Practice Guideline.

27. S. Bigos, "Understanding Acute Low Back Problems," AHCPR Quick Reference Guide.

28. D.C. Cherkin et al., "International Comparison."

29. N. Bogduk, "The Anatomical Basis for Spinal Pain Syndrome," Paper presented at the conference proceedings of the Chiropractic Centennial Foundation, Washington D.C., July 6-8, 1995.

30. J.F. Bourdillon and E.A. May, *"Spinal Manipulation,"* in *William Heinemann Medical Books,* 4th ed. (Norwalk, Conn.: Appleton and Lange, 1987), 203.

31. *Ibid.*

32. H. Rosomoff, "The Chiropractic Report," ed. David Chapman-Smith, 2 (5), July 1988.

33. Pran Manga, "Chiropractic Management."

34. S. Bigos, "Acute Problems in Adults," AHCPR Quick Reference Guide.

35. C. Pedersen, "Management of Spasticity on Neurophysiological Basis," *Scandinavian Journal of Rehabilitation Medicine.*

36. G. Waddell, "Modern Management."

37. S.H. Roth, *Drugs* 40(5S): 25-28 (1990).

38. "AMA Pocket Guide to Back Pain" (Random House, 1995).

39. T.S. Carey et al., "The Outcomes and Costs of Care for Acute Low Back Pain among Patients seen by Primary Care Practitioners, Chiropractors, and Orthopedic Surgeons," *NEJM* 333.(4).

40. B.W. Koes et al., "Randomized Clinical Trial of Manipulative Therapy and Physiotherapy for Persistent Back and Neck Complaints: Results of One Year Follow Up," *British Medical Journal,* 304 (7 March 1992): 601-605.

41. K.B. Jarvis et al., "Cost per Case Comparison of Back Injury Claims of Chiropractic versus Medical Management for Conditions with Identical Diagnostic Codes," *Journal of Occupational Medicine,* 33 (8): 847-52 (Aug. 1991).

42. S. Wolk, "Chiropractic versus Medical Care: A Cost Analysis of Disability and Treatment for Back-Related Workers' Compensation Cases," *FCER* September 1988.

43. L.G. Schifrin, "Mandated Health Insurance Coverage for Chiropractic Treatment: An Economic Assessment with Implications for the Commonwealth of Virginia," (The College of William and Mary, Williamsburg, Va., and the Medical College of Virginia, Richmond, Va., Jan 1992).

44. D.H. Dean and R.M. Schmidt, "A Comparison of the Costs of Chiropractors versus Alternative Medical Practitioners," (University of Richmond, Va., January 1992).

45. "Back Pain Sufferers Are Often Unsuspecting Recipients of Dangerous, Experimental Spinal Implants," "Public Citizen" news release, Washington, D.C., December 20, 1994.

46. *Ibid.*

47. S. Bigos, "Acute Problems in Adults," AHCPR Clinical Practice Guideline.

48. Ruth Jackson, *The Cervical Syndrome.*

49. *Ibid.*

50. S. Bigos, "Acute Problems in Adults," AHCPR Clinical Practice Guideline.

51. Juergen Kraemer, *Spine* 20(6):635-9 (1995).

Chapter Four

1. J.L. Shaw, "The Role of the Sacroiliac Joints as a Cause of Low Back Pain and Dysfunction," Speech before World Congress on Low Back Pain, University of California, San Diego, November 5-6, 1992.

2. Floyd Gilles, "Infantile Atlanto-Occiptal Instability - Potential Dangers of Extreme Extension," *Am. J. Dis. Child* 133 (1979).

3. R.A. Deyo, "Back Pain: The Best Treatment is Surprisingly Simple," *Consumer Reports*, September 1995.

4. Wilk v. AMA, testimony of J. M. Mennell, May 6, 1987.

5. *Ibid.*

6. B. Pettibone, seminar notes.

7. Juergen Kraemer, *Spine* 20(6): 635-9 (1995).

8. "The Backletter," 10(7): 73-83, (1995)..

9. G. Plaugher et al. "A Retrospective Consecutive Case Analysis of Pretreatment and Comparative Static Radiological Parameters Following Chiropractic Adjustments," *Journal of Manipulative and Physiological Therapeutics* 13(9): 498-506 (1990).

10. G.A. Tarola, "Manipulation for the Control of Back Pain and Curve Progression in Patients with Skeletally Mature Idiopathic Scoliosis: Two Case Studies," *Journal of Manipulative and Physiological Therapeutics* 17(4): 253-257 (1994).

11. C.A. Sallahian, "Reduction of Scoliosis in an Adult Male Utilizing Specific Chiropractic Spinal Manipulation: A Case Report," *The Journal of Chiropractic Research and Clinical Investigation* 7(2): 42-45 (1991).

12. A. Gamble, "Alternative Medical Approaches to the Treatment of Asthma," *Alternative and Complementary Therapies* 1(2): 61-66 (1995).

13. J.R. Jamison, A.P. McEwen and S.J. Thomas, "Chiropractic Adjustment in the Management of Visceral Conditions: A Critical Approach. *Journal of Manipulative and Physiological Therapeutics* 15(3): 171-180 (1992).

14. P.S. Ebrall, "Descriptive Report of the Case-Mix Within Australian Chiropractic Practice, 1992," *Chiropractic Journal of Australia* 23(3): 92-97 (1993).

15. D.H. Lines, "A Wholistic Approach to the Treatment of Bronchial Asthma in a Chiropractic Practice," *Chiropractic Journal of Australia* 23(1): 4-8 (1993).

16. D. Dennis and D. Golden, "Manipulative Therapy, An Alternative Treatment for Asthma: A Literature Review," *The Journal of Chiropractic Research and Clinical Investigation* 8(2): 40-41 (1992).

17. N. Klougart, N. Nilsson and J. Jacobsen, "Infantile Colic Treated by Chiropractors: A Prospective Study of 316 Cases," *Journal of Manipulative and Physiological Therapeutics* 17(4): 281-288 (1989).

18. W.R. Reed, S. Beavers, S.K. Reddy and G. Kern, "Chiropractic Management of Primary Nocturnal Enuresis," *Journal of Manipulative and Physiological Therapeutics* 17(9): 596-600 (1994).

19. M.A. Schmidt, "Otitis Media in Children," *Journal of Naturopathic Medicine* 5(1): 17-26 (1994).

20. B.F. Degenhardt and M.L. Kuchera, "Efficacy of Osteopathic Evaluation and Manipulative Treatment in Reducing the Morbidity of Otitis Media in Children," *Journal of the American Osteopathic Association* 94(8): 673 (1994).

21. J. Wadsworth and A.G. Chila, "Temporalis Muscle and Fascia in Relation to Otitis

Media," *Journal of the American Osteopathic Association* 94(8): 678 (1994).

22. T. Lehnert, "Acute Otitis Media in Children: Role of Antibiotic Therapy," *Canadian Family Physician* 39: 2157-2162 (1993).

23. L.C. Kleinman, J. Kosecoff, R.W. Dubois and R.H. Brook, "The Medical Appropriateness of Tympanostomy Tubes Proposed for Children Younger Than 16 Years in the United States," *Journal of the American Medical Association* 271(16): 1250-1255 (1994).

24. B.D. Inglis, "Chiropractic in New Zealand: Report of the Commission of Inquiry into Chiropractic," (Wellington, New Zealand, Government Printer, 1979).

25. Pran Manga et al., "Chiropractic Management."

26. S. Bigos, "Acute Problems in Adults," AHCPR Clinical Practice Guideline.

27. Ruth Jackson, *The Cervical Syndrome.*

28. A. Kleynhans, "Complications of and Contraindications to Spine Manipulative Therapy," in *Modern Developments in the Principles and Practice of Chiropractic,* ed. Scott Haldeman (New York: Appleton Century Crafts, 1980).

29. Philip Lee, News Release on AHCPR Guideline on Low Back Pain In Adults, U.S. Public Health Service, DHHS, December 8, 1994.

30. J. Jentzen, News Release, AHCPR Guideline on Low Back Pain in Adults, December 8, 1994.

31. D.M. Cloud and D. Ingram, *Goucester County Times,* March 13, 1994.

32. Edward Handley, AP news article, December 9, 1994.

33. "FCER News Alert," 2: January 1995.

34. Lowry R. Morton, Press conference on release of AHCPR Guideline on Low Back Pain in Adults, December 8, 1994.

35. "MDs CANNOT Perform Chiropractic Manipulation Rules Kansas Atty. General," *Dynamic Chiropractic* 14(7):1 (March 25, 1996).

36. M. Meyer et al., "A Pain for Business. Strain injuries: Will the Feds Crack Down?" *Newsweek* (June 28, 1995): 42.

Chapter Five

1. P. Joseph Lisa, *The Assault on Medical Freedom,* (Norfolk Va.: Hamptoms Roads, 1994).

2. M. Anthony, *Australian Family Physician,* November 1994.

3. H.T. Vernon, "Spinal Manipulation and Headaches of Cervical Origin: A Review of Literature and Presentation of Cases," *J Man Med* 6 (1991): 73-79.

4. J.S. Wight, "Migraine: A Statistical Analysis of Chiropractic Treatment," *J Am Chiropr Assoc* 12 (1978): 363-367.

5. G.B. Parker, D.S. Pryor, and H.A. Tupling, "A Controlled Trial of Cervical Manipulation for Migraine," *Aust NZ J Med* 8 (1978): 598-593.

6. J.M. Droz and F. Crot, "Occipital Headaches: Statistical Results in the Treatment of Vertebragenous Headache," *Annals Swiss Chirop Assoc* 8 (1985): 127-136.

7. Z. Turk and O. Ratkolb, "Mobilization of the Cervical Spine in Chronic Headaches," *J. Man Med* 3 (1987):15-17.

8. J. Stodolny and H. Chmielewshi, "Manual Therapy in the Treatment of Patients with Cervical Migraine," *J. Man Med* 4 (1989): 49-51.

9. P.D. Boline and C. Nelson, "Chiropractic and Pharmaceutical Therapy: A Randomized Clinical Trial for the Treatment of Chronic Muscle Contraction Headache," Proceedings of the FCER International Conference on Spinal Manipulation, Washington DC, 177-180 (1991).

10. P. Rothbart, *Toronto Star* Life Section, (December 28, 1995): 1.

11. W.O. Spitzer, "Scientific Approach to the Assessment and Management of Activity-Related Spinal Disorders: A Monograph for Clinicians," *Spine* 12 (suppl. S1-S59).

12. Floyd Gilles, "Infantile Atlanto-Occiptal Instability."

13. Abraham Towbin, "Latent Spinal Cord and Brain Stem Injury in Newborn Infants," *Develop. Med. Child Neurol.* 11 (1969): 54-68.

14. L. Spigelblatt et al., "The Use of Alternative Medicine," *Journal of Pediatrics* 94(1994)::811-14.

15. *American Journal of Public Health*, April 1992.

16. D.R. Mierau and J.D. Cassidy, "Sacroiliac Joint Dysfunction and Low Back Pain in School Aged Children," *JMPT*, 1984.

17. M.O. Tortti, J.J. Salminen, H.E. Paajanen, P.H. Terho, and M.J. Kormano, "Low-Back Pain and Disc Degeneration in Children: A Case-Control MR Imaging Study," Dept. of Diagnostic Radiology, Univ. of Turku, Finland. *Radiology* (August 1991) 180 (2): 503-7.

18. M.O. Erkintalo, J.J. Saliminen, A.M. Alanen, H.E. Paajanen, M.J. Kormano, "Development of Degenerative Changes in the Lumbar Intervertebral Disc: Results of a Prospective MR Imaging Study in Adolescents With and Without Low-Back Pain," Dept. of Diagnostic Radiology, Univ. of Turku, Finland. *Radiology* (August 1995) 196 (2): 529-33.

19. P. Shekelle, "20/20," ABC News Program, 1992.

20. P. Shelkelle, "Good News for Bad Backs," *Reader's Digest*, May 1995, 119-123.

BIBLIOGRAPHY

Allan O.B., Waddell G. "A Historical Perspective on Low Back Pain and Disability." *Acta Orthop Scand* 60 (1989) Suppl 234.

Back Pain: Report of a CSAG Committee on Back Pain, Clinical Standards Advisory Group, National Health Service, London, England, May 1994.

Bigos S, Bowyer O, Braen G, et al. *Acute Low Back Problems in Adults, Clinical Practice Guideline No. 14*. AHCPR Publication No. 95-0642. Rockville, MD: Agency for Health Care Policy and Research, Public Health Service, U.S. Department of Health and Human Services, December 1994.

Bogduk, N, MD, PhD. "The Anatomical Basis for Spinal Pain Syndrome." Paper presented at the Conference Proceedings of the Chiropractic Centennial Foundation, Washington D.C., July 1995.

Bourdillon, JF and EA May. (1987) *Spinal Manipulation*. 4th ed. Norwalk Ct/Los Altos, Ca. Appleton and Lange.

Cherkin DC, Deyo RA, Loeser JD, Bush T, Waddell G. "An International Comparison of Back Surgery Rates." *Spine* 19, no. 11 (1994): 1201-1206.

Cherkin, DC, MacCornack FA, "Patient Evaluation of Low Back Pain Care from Family Physicians and Chiropractors." *West J. Med.*, 150 (March 1989):351-355.

Croft, AC, DC, and SM Foreman, DC. *Whiplash Injuries - The cervical acceleration/deceleration syndrome*. Williams & Wilkins, 1988.

Davis H., "Increasing Rate of Cervical and Lumbar Spine Surgery in the United States, 1979-1990" *Spine* 19, no. 10: 1117-1124.

Dean DH and RM Schmidt. "A Comparison of the Costs of Chiropractors versus Alternative Medical Practitioners," University of Richmond, Va., 13 Jan. 1992.

DHEW Publ, #76-998 (NIH), "The Research Status of Spinal Manipulative Therapy."

Ebrall PS. "Mechanical Low-Back Pain: A Comparison of Medical and Chiropractic Management Within the Victorian WorkCare Scheme." *Chiropractic Journal of Australia*, vol. 22, # 2 (June 1992): 47-53.

Eisenberg DM et al. "Unconventional Medicine in the United States", *New England Journal of Medicine*, vol 328, no. 4, (28 Jan. 1993): 246-252.

Gallup Organization. "Demographic Characteristics of Users of Chiropractic Services." Princeton, N.J., 1991.

Hawk, C, LZ Killinger, and ME Dusio. "Perceived Barriers to Chiropractic Utilization: Qualitative Study Using Focus Groups." *Journal of the American Chiropractic Association*, vol. 32, no. 6 (June 1995): 39-44.

Jackson, R, MD. *The Cervical Syndrome*. 4th edition. Springfield, Ill., Charles C. Thomas, 1977.

Jarvis KB, et al. "Cost per Case Comparison of Back Injury Claims of Chiropractic versus Medical Management for Conditions with Identical Diagnostic Codes," *Journal of Occupational Medicine*, vol. 33, no. 8, (August 1991):

847-52.

Jensen MC, et al. "Magnetic Resonance Imaging of the Lumbar Spine in People Without Back Pain." *New England Journal of Medicine* vol. 331, no. 2 (1994):60-73.

Joseph, LP. *The Assault on Medical Freedom.* Norfolk, Va.: Hamptoms Roads, 1994.

Koes, BW et al. "Randomized Clinical Trial of Manipulative Therapy and Physiotherapy for Persistent Back and Neck Complaints: Results of One Year Follow Up," *British Medical Journal,* vol. 304 (7 March 1992): 601-605.

Manga, P et al., "The Effectiveness and Cost-Effectiveness of Chiropractic Management of Low-Back Pain", Ontario Ministry of Health, 1993.

Meade, TW et al. "Low Back Pain of Mechanical Origin: Randomized Comparison of Chiropractic and Hospital Outpatient Treatment." *British Medical Journal,* vol. 300 #67137 (2 June 1990): 1431-1437.

Mennell, JM, MD, testimony in the U.S. District Court, Northern District of Illinois, May 6, 1987, before the Honorable Susan Getzendanner.

Mushinski, M. "Average Hospital Charges for Medical and Surgical Treatment of Back Problems: United States, 1993", *Statistical Bulletin,* Metropolitan Life Insurance Company, Health and Safety Education Division, Medical Department, April-June 1995.

Nachemson, A. "Low Back Pain. Are Orthopedic Surgeons Missing the Boat?" *Acta Orthop Scand* 64 no. 1 (1993):1-2.

National Center for Health Statistics. Vital Health Statistics. "Detailed Diagnoses and Procedures, National Hospital Discharge Survey, 1990." (1992), by EJ Graves, 13, no. 13.

Payer, L. *Disease-Mongers.* John Wiley & Sons, 1992.

Shekelle, PG et al., "The Appropriateness of Spinal Manipulation for Low-Back Pain." RAND Corporation Report, Santa Monica, Calif., 1992.

Schifrin, LG. "Mandated Health Insurance Coverage for Chiropractic Treatment: An Economic Assessment with Implications for the Commonwealth of Virginia." The College of William and Mary and the Medical College of Virginia, Richmond, Va., January 1992.

Towbin, A. "Latent Spinal Cord and Brain Stem Injury in Newborn Infants", *Develop. Med. Child Neurol.* 11, (1969): 54-68.

U.S. Department of Defense. OCHAMPUS. "Chiropractic Evaluation Study Task III Report of the Relevant Literature." (24 January 1986), by MJ MacDonald and L Morton. Aurora, Colo.: MRI Project #8533-D.

Wolk, S. "Chiropractic versus Medical Care: A Cost Analysis of Disability and Treatment for Back-Related Workers' Compensation Cases." *FCER* (September 1988).

Zdeblick, TA. "A Prospective, Randomized Study of Lumbar Fusion - Preliminary Results." *Spine* 18 no. 8 (1993):983-991.

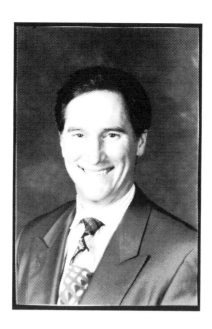

About the Author

𝒥.𝒞. 𝒮mith, DC, is a man of diverse interests. Growing up in southern California, he excelled in sports in high school, achieving All-American status in track as well as All-County at two positions in football. He also graduated from high school as a national merit scholar, which earned him an academic-athletic scholarship from the University of California at Berkeley. At Cal, he excelled at track again and was named to the 1968 All-American team. He also played varsity football and earned his B. S. degree in Conservation of Natural Resources.

After graduating from Cal and before beginning a three-year teaching/coaching stint at Rutgers University, Dr. Smith worked as a professional river guide on numerous white-water rivers throughout the West for four years. While at Rutgers, he earned his Masters in the Sociology of Sport from Goddard College in Cambridge, Mass. After his teaching experience at Rutgers, he enrolled in chiropractic college and graduated with honors in 1978.

Dr. Smith is married to Megan Hutnick, has four children and lives in a small town in middle Georgia, where he has practiced since 1980. He has a large menagerie of pets, keeps a flower garden, works out regularly, writes numerous articles, books, and health brochures, all the while operating a large chiropractic practice – one of only a few nationally certified spinal rehab facilities in the nation. In July 1996, Dr. Smith was the keynote speaker at the American Chiropractic Association's Council of Sports & Physical Fitness in Atlanta before the Olympic Festival in Atlanta.

If you have any inquiries about topics discussed in this book or seek further advice about your back problem, feel free to write Dr. Smith at his office: 1103 Russell Parkway, Warner Robins, GA. 31088.